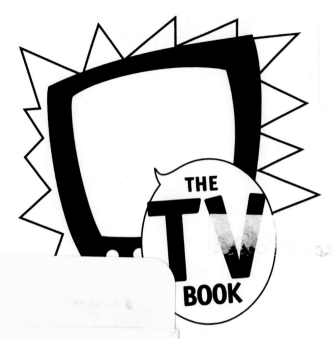

THE TV BOOK

o Your TV

gh Wallace

son and Brian Bean

ris M. Worsnop

Annick Press Ltd.
Toronto • New York • Vancouver

For my parents, Jack and Moira Wallace, who taught me that it was necessary, and fun, to talk back to TV, and for my husband, Jock Sutherland, who supported and encouraged me despite many hours of tuning in.
S.W.

©1996 Shelagh Wallace (text)
©1998 Shelagh Wallace (revised text)
©1996 Lorraine Tuson and Brian Bean (art)
©1998 Chris M. Worsnop (activities guide)
Project editor: Debora Pearson
Design: Brian Bean
Cover design: Sheryl Shapiro
Cover photo: Simon Shapiro

Annick Press Ltd.

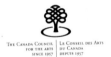
We acknowledge the support of the Canada Council for the Arts for our publishing program. We also thank the Ontario Arts Council.

THE CANADA COUNCIL | LE CONSEIL DES ARTS
FOR THE ARTS | DU CANADA
SINCE 1957 | DEPUIS 1957

Cataloguing in Publication Data
Wallace, Shelagh, 1960-
    The TV book : talking back to your TV

Rev. ed.
Includes index.
ISBN 1-55037-534-2

1. Television broadcasting – Social aspects – Juvenile literature. I. Worsnop, Chris. II. Tuson, Lorraine. III. Bean, Brian. IV. Title.

PN1992.57.W37 1998   j302.23'45   C98-930312-8

YA-
The text was typeset in Janson Text, Humanist 521, Runic, Univers 55 and Carta.

80140

Distributed in Canada by:
Firefly Books Ltd.
3680 Victoria Park Avenue
Willowdale, ON
M2H 3K1

Published in the U.S.A. by:
Annick Press (U.S.) Ltd.
Distributed in the U.S.A. by:
Firefly Books (U.S.) Inc.
P.O. Box 1338
Ellicott Station
Buffalo, NY 14205

Printed in Hong Kong.

Table of Contents

Introduction

When television was first introduced in North America over 50 years ago, some people predicted that it wouldn't last. After all, who would want to watch a fuzzy, little, black-and-white moving picture on a five-inch screen? Well, a lot of people, as it turned out, and nobody was more surprised than the owners of movie theatres and radio stations. By the early 1950s, movie theatres and restaurants were empty on Monday and Tuesday nights: people were staying home to watch Milton Berle and *I Love Lucy*. Today, a billion people around the world watch television. Watching TV is, in fact, what North Americans of all ages spend the most time doing, after sleeping and working or going to school. Recent studies show that North American kids watch an average of 18 to 26 hours of television a week. That's close to four hours a day – almost as much time as you spend daily at school.

And what's wrong with watching TV? You've probably heard some of the arguments: it cuts into the time you could spend reading, shortens your attention span, teaches bad habits, and causes you to grow fat from too much sitting around. Some people also criticize it for presenting "perfect" people and encouraging viewers to feel that they should be just as "perfect," even when that's impossible. Other people criticize TV for the opposite reason: they believe that showing not-so-nice people on TV gives viewers the mistaken idea that it's okay to be unpleasant, mean, and, in some cases, even violent.

Television is an important part of many people's lives, and this book will look at some of the ways that it touches you and affects your life. It will also help you discover some things that you may not already know, including who decides which series get on TV and what advertisers are, and aren't, allowed to do. And it will show you how *you* can have an effect on what you see on TV by communicating directly with the television networks – as you're about to find out, you (and other kids like you) are a very important part of the TV audience.

To help you develop your understanding of TV, we've included activities you can try and amazing facts, plus behind-the-scenes interviews with some

TV tidbit

According to a poll published in the June 1992 issue of *TV Guide,* one out of every four Americans claim that they wouldn't trade their TV sets for one million dollars. And in another survey conducted in the United States, kids were asked which they would keep if forced to make a choice between their fathers and their TV sets. The results? Over half of the kids chose their TVs!

unusual people, including kids, who are involved with TV. At the back of the book, we've listed the names and addresses of television networks, govern-

TV around the world

There are one billion television sets in the world. What are people watching on them?

- On evening TV in India, viewers can watch children reciting poetry that they have composed themselves. The most popular soap opera is *Same Search Again,* the story of a poor young man and a rich young woman who fall in love. And many Indians watch a talk show called *The Pritish Nandi Show.* It's hosted by a poet/magazine editor who interviews Indian rap singers and other celebrities.

- Russians are also big soap opera fans: the most popular TV show that ever aired in Russia was a Mexican soap opera called *The Rich Also Cry,* the story of a rich and powerful man who marries his beautiful maid. Russian viewers also love Russian game shows, music videos, and broadcasts from the parliament. In fact, when the Russian government first aired a daily broadcast of its parliament in 1989, people were so interested that they stayed home from work to watch it!

- In Israel, viewers have their choice of three stations from Germany, two from France, three from Turkey, and one each from Spain, Italy, Saudi Arabia, Jordan, and Egypt. Televised news is broadcast in five languages – Russian, French, Arabic, Hebrew, and English – and, unlike North American half-hour or hour-long newscasts, Israeli newscasts last as long as it takes to present the day's news.

- Ten years ago in China, there was only one station available to viewers. Today, Central Chinese Television (CCTV) has more than 500 stations and, in a country with a population of 1.1 billion people, the biggest audience in the world. In China, more viewers tune in to the news than any other TV program.

ment offices, and citizens' groups that you can write to in order to let them know what you think about what you see on TV, good or bad. Just as with the programs you watch, you can follow this book through from beginning to end or spend time on the sections that interest you the most. Either way, we hope you'll come back to *The TV Book* again and again.

This book is just a starting point: it doesn't cover everything about TV. (For instance, it doesn't deal with who invented the first television set or how TV signals make their way to your set.) *The TV Book* aims to start you thinking about the TV you watch in new ways and really "see" what's on TV. So, as you read this book, talk about television and what you see on it with your friends, parents, and teachers. Ask questions, watch carefully, think about what you see, and talk back to your TV.

Colour or black-and-white?

In a 1997 study, researchers counted the number of white people and people of colour in over 172 TV shows that kids 12 and under watch. (The shows the researchers included are programs made for kids and families that are shown during early weekday mornings, after school, and early evenings.) The researchers found that, out of every 100 main characters, more than 50 are white, about 12 are African-American, and only 10 are Asian, Latino, or Middle Eastern. The remainder are unidentifiable. When non-white characters do play central characters on TV, their roles are often negative stereotypes (for example, Arabs being shown as terrorists or other "bad guys").

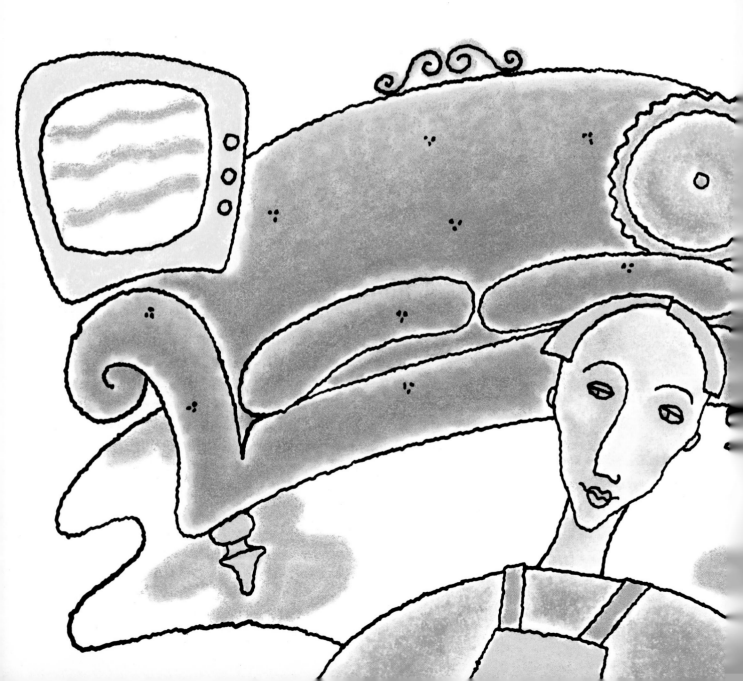

TV Land!

You're about to enter TV Land – that familiar, yet oh-so-unusual place where TV characters live. You've got the couch to yourself, the cushions just right, and sole control of the remote. As you surf through dozens of channels, you are able to identify, in just seconds, the different kinds of programs that are on. Wait a minute – how do you do all of that so fast?

Tune in to the Details

You, along with millions of other TV viewers, understand what you see on TV because it uses "conventions": widely recognized details and ways of doing things that you accept and understand as being part of particular TV shows. Conventions help you quickly tell what's going on, and that's important – after you take out the commercials, half-hour programs have only 22 minutes to tell a story, and hour-long programs have just 48 minutes.

Of course, when you're watching TV, the conventions are so familiar that you don't notice them. But what happens if you listen to the TV with your eyes closed? Just by listening, you'll recognize some shows by some of their particular details and ways of doing things. You'll pick out a comedy by the audience's laughter, a drama by its suspenseful music and the actors' solemn tones, and a game show by the announcer's voice and the constant bells and buzzers.

Now what happens when you mute the sound and just watch the screen? You'll still recognize a comedy, even if you can't hear the laughter, because the action is usually confined to a couple of brightly lighted sets, often in the family home and usually the living room. A drama has more sets, and more natural lighting. Other shows have completely different conventions than either a comedy or a drama. A news show, for example, has carefully groomed

Where are all the girls in TV land?

In a 1997 study, researchers counted the number of males and females on kids' and family shows on the major American networks, PBS, and cable networks. They discovered that only 35 percent of the main characters on these shows are female.

anchors who sit behind a desk.

Some TV shows use certain conventions to make you think you're watching a particular kind of show when you're actually not. For example, "tabloid" programs like *Hard Copy* and *Inside Edition* look like regular newscasts, with their anchors at a desk, but they present stories that are sometimes more entertainment than fact. And some made-for-TV movies that are based on real events depend

TV talk

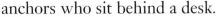

The word "television" comes from the Greek words "tele," which means "from a distance," and "vision," which means "to see." It first appeared in *Scientific American* magazine in 1907. Since then, words to do with television have become an important part of our language. Can you match each TV expression on the left with its correct meaning on the right? Then check your answers on page 95.

1. idiot box   a. a person who can't seem to watch one show at a time

2. channel surfer   b. what you use to zip through channels

3. sofa spud   c. what people might call you if you spend too much time sitting in front of the TV

4. zapper   d. along with "squawk box," it's a nickname for television

Is it real or is it entertainment?

Back in the 1950s, quiz shows were the most popular nighttime TV shows. Fans loved shows like *Treasure Hunt* and *Strike It Rich* because they supposedly put ordinary people in situations where they could win huge amounts of money. Contestants on shows such as *Twenty-One* and *The $64,000 Question* became especially famous because they answered incredibly difficult questions week after week. But in 1959, during congressional hearings in the States, the truth about the quiz shows came out. Herbert Stempel, a former quiz show champ, testified that the producers of *Twenty-One* and *The $64,000 Question* decided ahead of time which contestant would win each night, and which would lose. Contestants were given both the questions and the answers before the show and told how to act as if they were struggling with the answers. TV viewers were shocked: they had believed that the contestants were behaving honestly and that the winners were the people who answered correctly on the spot. The shows' producers acted on the assumption that quiz shows were just entertainment – after all, no one minded if things were made up in TV dramas or comedies. All the big quiz shows were taken off the air, and in 1960 the government made it a federal crime to "fix" game shows, or decide the outcome in advance. It wasn't until 1972 that most of the game shows were allowed to return to TV.

Deception remains a problem today. Despite tabloid talk-show hosts claiming their guests are authentic, there have been many reports that actors are hired to play some of the more outrageous guests.

on conventions from drama shows. The exciting music and interesting settings help make the movie more interesting to watch than it would be if the events were shown the way they actually happened.

Meet Some Very Familiar Faces

Like conventions, standard character types, or "stereotypes," are used on TV because viewers quickly and easily recognize them. For instance, as soon as you see an awkward character with weird clothes and glasses, you instantly assume that this character is smart but nerdy. The show's writers don't need to spend a lot of time explaining that he or she is rather clever at school but uncomfortable with people. You've probably seen other TV Land stereotypes, such as the goofy best friend who causes problems; the all-knowing, always understanding parents; the annoying little sister or brother; the ugly bad guy; and the dumb blonde. Stereotyped TV characters are entertaining to watch because they're such obvious exaggerations of certain kinds of

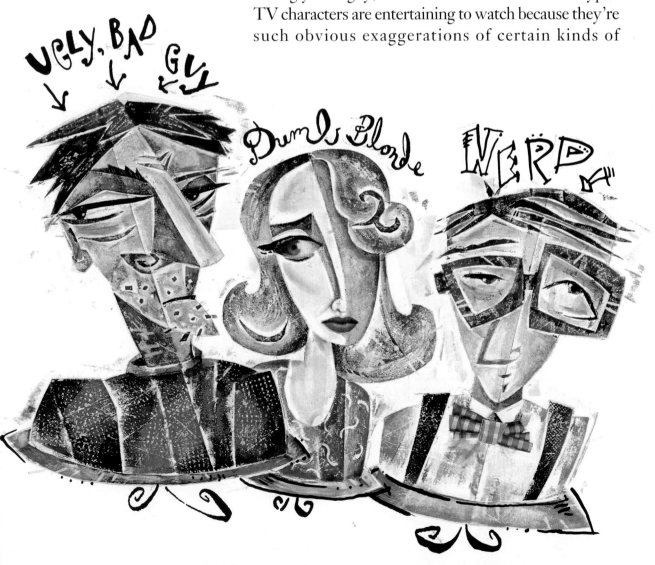

UGLY, BAD GUY

Dumb Blonde

NERD

people. On the other hand, most stereotypes aren't at all like people in real life – is there a stereotyped character in TV Land that is similar to you and just as interesting and complex as you are?

Conventions and stereotypes are so much fun to watch that you usually accept them and don't question what you are shown. That's true of other things you see in TV Land as well. In fact, if you watch a lot of TV, you probably accept certain things you see on television as being true, even though they are not. A Pennsylvania researcher named George Gerbner discovered this when he asked people who watched a lot of TV (more than four hours a day) and a little TV (less than two hours a day) some questions, including the one below. See what your answer is, then compare it to the answers that the "heavy" TV viewers gave George Gerbner.

What are your chances of being a crime victim during this next year?

a) one in a million b) one in fifty c) one in ten

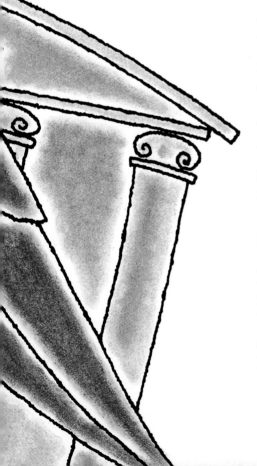

TV tidbit

According to newspaper reports, at a May, 1994 conference about TV sponsored by the American cable network CNN, a Sarawak Indian from Malaysia spoke about the effects of TV on his people. He said that since the young people of his tribe started watching World Championship Wrestling they had stopped honouring their elders and started idolizing wrestlers such as "Nature Boy" Ric Flair instead.

People who watch a lot of TV usually believe that they have a high chance of being a victim of crime and so they choose c), or a one in ten chance. That's because crime on TV happens a lot more often than it does in real life – ten times as often! You actually only have a one in fifty chance of being a victim of crime next year.

People who watch a lot of TV also believe that lawyers are always in the courtroom trying criminals, while, in real life, only some lawyers ever see the inside of a courtroom. Heavy TV viewers also think that the police fire their guns a lot because on TV a cop kills up to 50 people a year. A real-life police officer uses his or her gun far less often – on average, once every 27 years.

More female than male characters are victims of TV violence. And while young males aren't usually the characters hurt on TV, in real life they are the group most likely to be hurt or killed through involvement with violence.

It All Happens So Fast

Life in TV Land often seems more exciting and interesting than real life. In TV Land, the boring bits of life are left out. TV Land kids don't usually spend hours doing their homework, watching TV, or lying around on the couch staring into space the way you or your friends might. And any problems that come up are usually resolved within the half-hour or one-hour time slot. (Don't you wish things were really like that?) Things happen quickly in TV Land, and that helps to hold your attention.

TV Jolts: They'll Grab Your Attention!

Television shows also hold your attention by "jolting" you with sudden actions, fast camera movements, heart-pumping music, and loud noises. If there aren't enough jolts per minute, or "jpms," TV producers think you're likely to switch channels. (Psychologists say it takes about six jpms to keep you glued to the set.) Even *Sesame Street* has a high jpm count: in an hour-long show, it may have 45 different

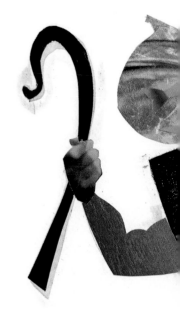

TV families get tough

If you watch a lot of TV sitcoms, you might get the impression that there is such a thing as the perfect family. TV Land families, especially those on sitcoms, are almost always healthy, attractive, and happy. But some popular sitcoms, such as *Roseanne* and *The Simpsons,* deliberately show families that aren't perfect. Are these TV Land families closer to what a real family is like? When *Parenting Magazine* asked its readers which television family was most similar to their own family, 40 percent said *Roseanne,* 28 percent said *Leave It to Beaver,* 7 percent said *The Simpsons,* and another 7 percent said *The Addams Family*!

segments, some as short as five seconds. Commercials often have even more jolts than the shows they interrupt. In 30 seconds, they can contain on average 10 to 15 changes from one shot to another, as well as special effects, flashy colours, and loud noise and music.

One of the most obvious differences between Canadian and American shows is that Canadian ones, on average, have fewer jolts per minute.

Remote controls have made it even more difficult and challenging for TV producers to keep viewers like you watching. In the days before remotes, you actually had to get up and cross the room to change channels. Now, if a show is even a little bit slow you can "click" to another program or turn off the set altogether.

Because of this, the people who make the shows have had to come up with new ways to keep you watching. They use "teasers," or commercials that promote the program coming up after the one you're watching, to tempt you to stay tuned. And, recently, some networks have removed the commercials between programs so that after you finish watching one show you immediately start watching the one that follows it. This happens so quickly that you usually don't have time to even think about changing channels. Television people call this the "hot switch."

So enjoy your next trip to TV Land and take a good look around while you're there – there's more to it than meets the eye!

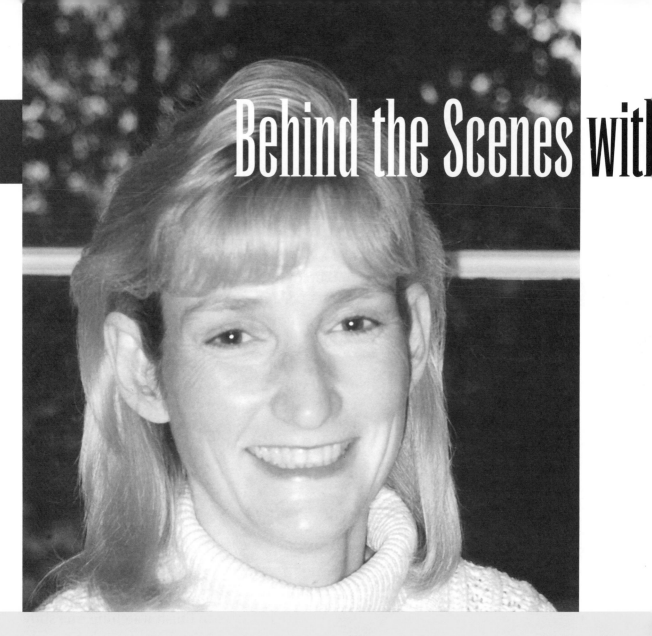

Lynne Carrow started out as an actor, but later discovered that what she really wanted to do was work behind the scenes. For three years, she was the casting director for the popular TV show *The X-Files*. These days she's casting parts for Sunday night's *Wonderful World of Disney* and a new CBC TV series called

Lynne Carrow

Interviewer: What does a TV casting director do?

Lynne: I'm hired by the producer and director of a TV show or series to help cast the actors. First, they give me the script and I read it. Then I break down the characters, which means I do a quick description of each character. Very often they aren't in the script and you have to figure things out by looking for clues.

Interviewer: Does the director help you figure out what each character is like?

Lynne: It hardly ever happens that they say, "Well, this is what I'm looking for in this character." A lot of the time, they don't know. So I look for all the clues I can find in the script, including the dialogue, and hope that I'm on the right track.

Interviewer: How many actors do you audition for each part?

Lynne: About five at the most. I like to bring in people with very different looks and different ethnic backgrounds. If the role isn't specifically for a male, I also bring in some women to audition for the part. I'm always trying to get the best actor and often the best one is a woman. So if I'm casting the role of a doctor and the doctor's name is Mark, it can be changed to Martine so that a woman can play the part. Most TV directors and producers are open to changing things like that, provided it isn't essential to the story that the doctor is a man.

Interviewer: What is "typecasting"?

Lynne: There's a lot of typecasting on TV. Part of typecasting has to do with an actor's appearance. Most actors can only play the characters that they look like or that we believe they look like. For instance, if you look like a bad guy, you're going to play a bad guy.

Interviewer: What does a bad guy look like?

Lynne: Acne scars on the face, crooked teeth — the stereotyped kind of things you might expect. If you notice, on TV now only the bad guys smoke. There's something sinister-looking about a bad guy's face, even though the person playing the bad guy might be the most gentle human on earth. I know several actors like that. I will bring them in to audition for the part of the nice dad, but they will be cast as the Mafia guy.

Interviewer: Why do you think that happens?

Lynne: During an episode of a dramatic TV series, you only have one hour minus commercials and you have to sell a character instantly. If someone comes on and he has only a few lines and he looks like a bad guy, you're not going to be able to convince viewers that he's the nice man next door. You need a more round-faced guy with dimples and twinkling blue eyes, so that as soon as viewers see him they say, "Yes, he's a good guy."

Interviewer: What other types of characters have you cast?

Lynne: I often had to cast the FBI type for *The X-*

Files. They were really easy to cast because they all looked exactly alike. They're fairly attractive, they're fit, and their faces are very normal. You can't have someone with a huge scar as an FBI type on TV, although in real life an FBI agent might have such a scar. But not on TV, unless there's a whole storyline about how the character got the scar. It looks too unusual.

Interviewer: Do you think that characters in TV shows should be more like real-life people?

Lynne: People don't want to watch real life on TV. For most shows to succeed, they have to be more interesting and more exciting than real life or they're really boring to watch. Take a TV movie based on a real-life story – the woman in the story may be fat and pimply in real life, but you can't show this on TV because nobody would watch her. Instead, the people who are doing the casting will turn the character into a more attractive person and cast a good-looking actress to play the role.

Interviewer: You've been a casting director for more than 15 years. Do you think the TV shows today are doing less typecasting than they used to?

Lynne: They're casting more against type with shows like *The X-Files* and other shows that imitate it. But I'd say that's the exception. That's why it was really fun to be the casting director for *The X-Files*. It was the biggest hit I've ever worked on and I got to find lots of weird people instead of mostly cops, which is what I would have had to do on other TV shows!

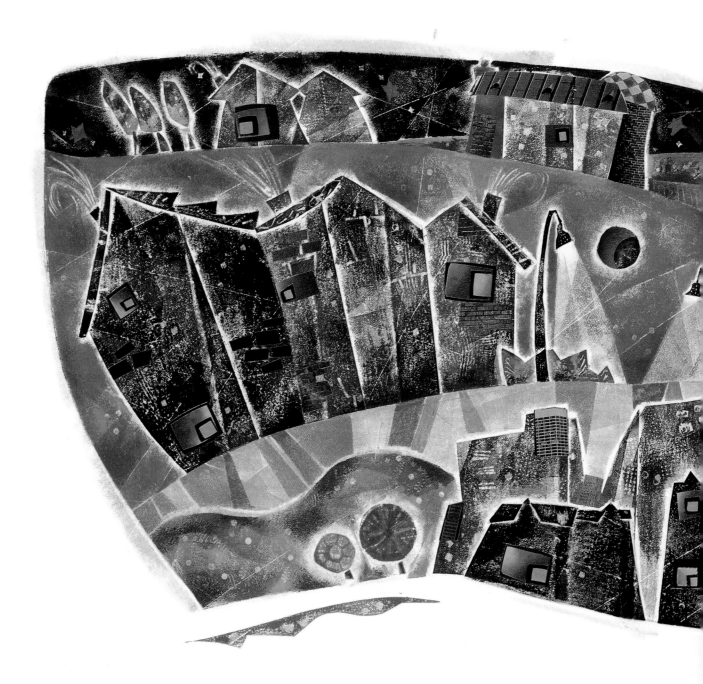

...d a TV Series

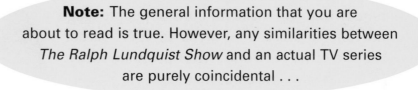

Note: The general information that you are about to read is true. However, any similarities between *The Ralph Lundquist Show* and an actual TV series are purely coincidental . . .

It's spring, and the latest Nielsen ratings from the February "sweeps," a month-long rating sweepstakes or survey when the American audience is carefully measured, show some bad news for network XYZ. It's running last among the networks in the race for ratings on Wednesday nights between 8 and 10 p.m. Only a small percentage of the people watching TV during that time are tuning in to XYZ shows.

The vice-presidents of programming at XYZ realize they must make some big changes to the Wednesday night lineup to win back the audience. They take two of XYZ's popular programs which air on other nights and move them to Wednesday night. They also decide to create a new series.

They Get the Idea

First, XYZ approaches TV producers and some well-known actors for their ideas about a new series. The producers and actors are told what XYZ is looking-for in a new series: a half-hour situation comedy that will make millions of people laugh and tune in week after week to XYZ rather than the other networks. Most program ideas never become series, but hundreds get to the first stage, the "pilot," or single trial episode, of a new show.

The famous TV star, Ralph Lundquist, has an idea. What about a TV show based on his life, starring him, produced by him, and called *The Ralph Lundquist Show*?

Time to Test It Out

It can cost about $1 million to produce a single pilot and XYZ wants to be certain, before it spends that much, that *The Ralph Lundquist Show* will be popular. Like other networks, XYZ hires market researchers to test series ideas long before the scripts are written, the actors are cast, and the pilot is taped. The researchers conduct "focus groups," in which people are recruited to form a sample audience. These people are given descriptions of the characters and stories and asked their opinions.

Ralph's show passes this testing with flying colours. The sample audience loves Ralph's adopted teenage son Emo, their chimpanzee named Zee, and

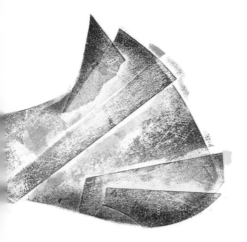

the Mexican setting. The audience doesn't like the idea of Ralph, Emo, and Zee involved in a bank robbery, but XYZ isn't worried: the story can be easily changed at this point.

The next step is to rewrite the story and test it again. The second sample audience unanimously approves of the new story about Ralph, Emo, and Zee running a hairdressing salon. The scripts are written, the actors are cast, and the pilot is taped.

It's your choice!

According to information gathered from ratings, most boys don't watch kids' TV shows with female lead characters. On the other hand, most girls will watch shows with either female or male lead characters. What about you – what do you prefer to watch?

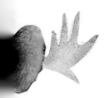

Test, Tests, and More Tests

Ralph's pilot is finally ready to be screened in front of more sample audiences. Viewers are invited to come to a hotel conference room to watch several half-hour shows, including *The Ralph Lundquist Show*, and some commercials. Then the viewers are given a list of questions to answer, including: How would you rate this show? Do you like the main character? Would you watch this show at 8 p.m. on Wednesday nights? The viewers are also asked what their age is, if they are male or female, and how much money they earn.

All the testing indicates that Ralph's show will be a big hit, but the decision on whether or not to turn it into a series rests with the XYZ vice-presidents of programming. They know that some pilots have tested brilliantly and then died in the ratings. Other pilots, for shows such as *Cheers*, *Family Ties*, and *Hill*

Street Blues, have tested miserably but have gone on to become popular series after they were given a second chance by network vice-presidents.

The vice-presidents look at the test results carefully. With which age groups was Ralph's show most popular? Did male and female viewers respond differently? Did viewers who made over forty thousand dollars a year like the show more than viewers who made less than forty thousand dollars? The market research indicates that Ralph's show will be most popular with both male and female viewers between the ages of 18 and 49. The vice-presidents are pleased: this is the best audience for a series to have

How can you help your favourite program stay on the air?

Uh-oh! You've just read in the newspaper that your favourite show is extremely low in the ratings and is in danger of being cancelled. What can you do? You can try writing a letter to the network that airs the show. In your letter, state that you like the show and want it to stay on the air. (See pages 93-4 for addresses.) Sometimes letter-writing can help save a show; other times it can't. In 1995, ABC cancelled *My So-Called Life* despite receiving thousands of letters. Why? *My So-Called Life* was so low in the ratings that ABC couldn't afford to keep producing it any longer: the episodes cost more to produce than ABC could make back by selling advertising time. But don't despair – letter-writing viewers have helped to save several shows from cancellation, including *Cagney & Lacey, Beauty and the Beast,* and *Designing Women.*

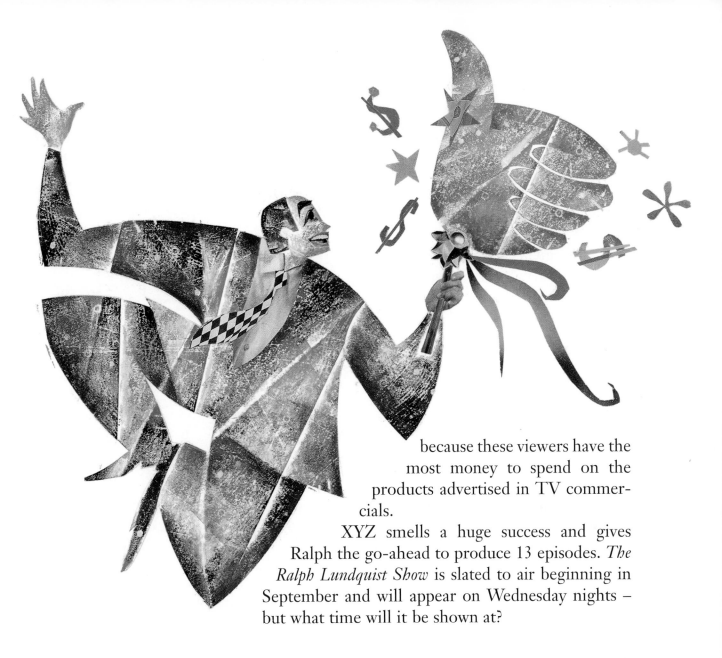

because these viewers have the most money to spend on the products advertised in TV commercials.

XYZ smells a huge success and gives Ralph the go-ahead to produce 13 episodes. *The Ralph Lundquist Show* is slated to air beginning in September and will appear on Wednesday nights – but what time will it be shown at?

It's about Time!

Scheduling, or finding the right time for a show, is very important. It's also very tricky. This show's target audience is made up mostly of adults who work during the day, so it is scheduled at night when the audience is home and likely to be watching TV. (Most people watch TV during the "prime-time" period, from 8 to 11 p.m. Monday through Saturday, and 7 to 11 p.m. on Sunday.) Finally the network decides: *The Ralph Lundquist Show* will air at 8:30 p.m.

The XYZ vice-presidents schedule the Wednesday night shows so that the extremely popular sitcom, *The Martin Tall Show*, will appear before Ralph at 8:00 p.m., giving it a strong lead-in. The two shows after Ralph's, at 9:00 p.m. and 9:30 p.m., are also popular sitcoms and have been moved here from other nights. The vice-presidents of programming have done what they can to ensure the success of Ralph's show: they've scheduled similar shows one after the other (counting on sitcom fans to stay tuned), and they've scheduled the new show between two popular shows.

The vice-presidents have also looked at what's being offered on the other networks and have tried to offer something different on XYZ. One network has a football game every Wednesday night and another shows an old movie. A block of four sitcoms on XYZ will attract a different audience than the either of the other networks get.

On with the Show!

During the summer, while Ralph and his crew are producing the episodes, staff from

TV networks around the world gather in Los Angeles to preview the new American shows and buy them for their own networks. Many of them find Ralph's show amusing. They gladly agree to pay the licensing fees that the producer demands so that they too may televise Ralph's show in their own countries.

The premiere of *The Ralph Lundquist Show* is set

MTV in India!

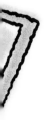 About half of the TV shows shown in countries outside of North America are made in the United States. Egyptians are hooked on the American soap opera *The Bold and the Beautiful,* while Europeans tune in to *Beverly Hills 90210* and *Baywatch.* In India MTV is a huge hit, and in China viewers follow *Little House on the Prairie.* Canadian programs are also popular. One show, *Ready or Not,* airs in 33 countries. Why are there so many North American shows in other countries?

It's usually cheaper for a foreign network to buy a North American show than it is for the same network to make its own program, even when the extra costs of translating the English dialogue and "dubbing," or adding a new soundtrack, are included. And American shows attract large foreign audiences, so the foreign networks that air them can charge more for advertising time and make more money than they would with other shows. But not every country welcomes U.S. TV shows. Some countries have established rules that restrict the number of American-made shows their country's stations can broadcast. France allows only 40 percent of its TV schedule to be American-made and Canada requires 50 percent of its prime-time programming to be Canadian. Japan has gone one step further: it broadcasts only programs produced in Japan. These countries believe that they have to protect their own unique culture by making sure that their TV viewers see shows made by their fellow citizens, about their own country.

Adults keep out!

Today, more than ever before, there are lots of TV shows made especially for kids. Many kids are big fans of both the shows and the kids' networks that produce and broadcast many of them. Geraldine Laybourne, former president of the U.S. kids' network Nickelodeon, believes that's because there's lots of pressure on kids to grow up too fast these days. She thinks that most of the "regular" networks add to that pressure by showing mainly adult programs. But kids' networks offer shows that focus on kids, are full of fun, and make kids feel respected and appreciated.

In the States, Nickelodeon reaches kids between the ages of two and fifteen in 60 million homes – that's more than ABC, NBC, and CBS combined. Nickelodeon broadcasts *Nick News*, a weekly newscast just for kids, and publishes a magazine, also called *Nickelodeon*, that's definitely *not* for adults.

In Canada, YTV (Youth Television Network) reaches kids, including "tweens" (nine- to fourteen-year-olds), in more than 6.8 million homes. Like Nickelodeon, YTV has a weekly news show that aims to entertain as well as inform kids. It also introduced Canadian audiences to young people known as program jockeys, or PJs, on its shows. Instead of commercials between shows, PJs read viewers' letters, describe contests kids can enter, tell stories, and just gab. "Regular" networks, also, are changing the way they've always done things to create television just for kids. They're discovering what Nickelodeon and YTV have known for years – that kids like you are an important part of the TV audience!

for Wednesday, September 15. All summer, XYZ has been advertising its arrival. Ralph has appeared on every TV talk show to present clips from the series and talk about it.

How Do They Rate?

Thursday morning, September 16: the overnight Nielsen ratings are in. The premiere of *The Ralph Lundquist Show* is a huge hit! It's the top-rated show, with a rating of 21, which means that 21% of the TV-watching households in the United States were watching Ralph's show. (Ratings are measured separately in the United States and Canada.)

Nielsen Media Research, the biggest company that measures North American TV audiences, gets the information for its Nielsen ratings in several different ways. To determine national ratings, researchers monitor TV use in more than 1,700 households in Canada and 9,000 in the U.S. with meters that are installed on TV sets, VCRs, and cable boxes, and attached to small computers and modems. The meters automatically track when the TV sets are on and which channel is being watched. Every night, that information is sent to Nielsen's central computers.

Nielsen also uses "People Meters," boxes about the size of a paperback that are attached to the TV set meters. Each family member is assigned their own button to push when they watch a TV program. The information collected from the People Meters lets the researchers know, for example, if more thirteen-year-olds than eight-year-olds are watching a particular program.

Ratings determine how much networks can charge advertisers for the commercials that appear during shows. The larger the audience, and the closer it is to the 18-to-49 group, the more money the networks can charge for advertising time. Advertising value is measured in CPMs (cost per one thousand TV viewers), so if the CPM is four dollars a minute and the show's audience is measured at two million homes, the cost of a 60-second commercial is eight thousand dollars!

Television advertising is sold a long time before a show appears on the air and before the network knows for certain how many people are watching it. XYZ guessed that *The Ralph Lundquist Show* would attract an audience of 15 million homes, based on the performance of similar sitcoms and the ratings for Wednesday nights in the past. The advertisers were happy because they ended up with a bargain: 19.6 million homes for the price of 15 million homes! (On the other hand, if Ralph's show hadn't attracted the size of audience it expected, the network would have had to give money back to the advertisers in free advertising. One network recently had to give back over twenty-five million dollars' worth of free advertising!)

Ralph Really Sweeps Up

Week after week, Ralph's program continues to place high in the ratings. And Ralph has planned some-

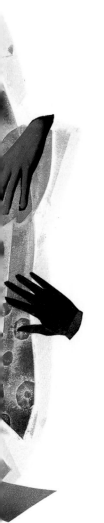

thing special for the November sweeps. Ratings sweepstakes, or "sweeps," take place four times a year and the networks go all-out to attract viewers. Zee has contracted a horrible disease and Ralph's friend, the TV star Ray Dart, is playing the doctor who must find the cure. The disease's discovery and its treatment will last throughout the four November episodes, which are expected to attract record audiences.

Sure enough, the November sweeps indicate that Ralph, Emo, and Zee are destined for TV stardom. The network asks for nine more episodes to complete the full season of 22 episodes. Ralph knows that only one out of five series gets renewed for a second year, but his show has remained high in the ratings – so far. If he can keep this up for another two years (a total of 66 episodes), as producer he can then lease, or syndicate, the series to the XYZ or other networks as a rerun. Rerun shows are broadcast repeatedly without any of the costs that go along with making new episodes – and that means that the money Ralph makes from syndicating his show will be pure profit!

Behind the Scenes wit

What's it like to be involved in the testing of TV shows? Just ask Goody Gerner –

she was the president and owner of Generations Research Incorporated, a

Toronto-based company that uses kids to test products, advertising ideas, and TV

shows. Goody and her company played an important role in helping make some

good TV shows even better!

oody Gerner

Interviewer: When you tested a kids' TV show, what did the network expect you to do?

Goody: It really depended on what stage the network was at with the show. Sometimes the show was at the idea stage, before they'd even shot anything, and we found out for them what kids thought about the idea. Sometimes we played the tapes of the actors who were auditioning for the show to see who kids liked the best. Other times, we'd test the rough cut of a TV pilot to find out what was working and what wasn't.

Interviewer: How did you find the kids who would be the "audience" and give you their opinions?

Goody: All kinds of ways. We put ads in newspapers, got referrals from people who had come to groups, names of friends, and things like that. We looked for kids who could think fast and who weren't shy about speaking out.

Interviewer: Did the kids get anything in return?

Goody: Yes, they were paid. The kids got anywhere from $30 to $40 Canadian.

Interviewer: What did you actually do when you were testing a show with some kids?

Goody: We usually tested with about five or six kids at a time. The kids came to a central location, usually a place that had a room with a one-way mirror. The people from the network and other people who were observing sat outside the room and looked through the mirror to see how the kids were reacting to the show. The kids inside the room couldn't see out through the mirror. I usually left the room and watched the kids through the mirror. If I were in the room with them, the kids would be on their best behaviour and watch the show that I put on. But if I left the room, they sometimes lost attention, made comments, and talked to someone else. It was important that we find out what their real response was.

Interviewer: Didn't the kids know that there were people on the other side of the mirror watching them?

Goody: Yes, you're required to tell them. But they forget, almost immediately. Adults forget too. Everybody forgets about the mirror!

Interviewer: How long did you do the testing for?

Goody: For no more than an hour. Kids can't sit longer than that. They just get antsy!

Interviewer: What kinds of questions did you ask?

Goody: Part of it depended on what we were testing. No matter what I was testing, I always asked them what did they like, what didn't they like, what was funny, dumb, cute, boring, exciting. I also asked who the show was most appropriate for – boys or girls? Kids older than you or younger than you? And I asked if they would want to watch the show again. Those kinds of things.

Interviewer: Do the networks look for specific answers to specific questions?

Goody: The networks may have specific things that they're concerned about. For instance, they might want to know how kids feel about the music or the show's set.

Interviewer: What happened after the testing?

Goody: During testing, each group was always audiotaped and sometimes videotaped, too. Afterward, the network could take the tapes away and study them. I wrote a report for the network which was my impressions of the testing. I backed up what I said in the report by including some of the kids' comments from the tapes.

Interviewer: If kids don't like a show, will a network rework it?

Goody: Yes.

Interviewer: How many times can a show go through this process?

Goody: I've tested the same show three or four times. Of the shows I've tested, most ended up on television because we helped make them better!

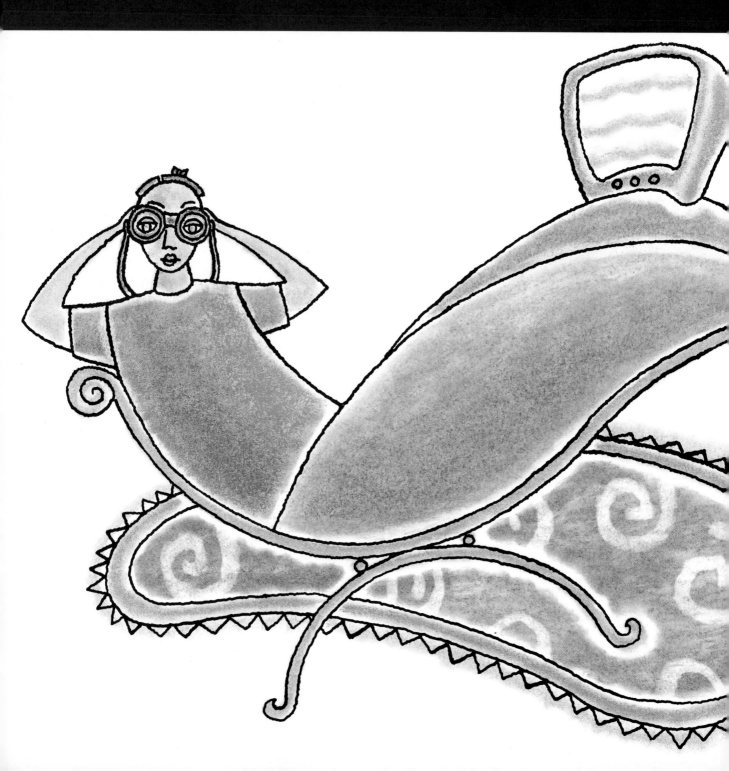

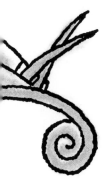

Look around the room you're in. Now, cup your hands around your eyes as though you're holding a pair of binoculars there. Look around the room again. As you look through the frame you've made with your cupped hands, you see only certain parts of the room at a time and you view them from your own unique position. You are seeing things from your point of view.

TV: A New Point of View

Like your cupped hands, a television screen frames what you see on TV and gives you a certain view of the show's sets, the actors, and the action. But unlike the things you see through your cupped hands, the pictures on your screen don't have your point of view. Instead, you're watching a point of view that was chosen by the show's directors (and then shot with cameras) to make you pay attention to the things that the directors have decided are important in the show. The directors also want you to react in specific ways to what you see – they want you to cheer the show's hero, but not the bad guy – and so they use a number of tricks to make this happen.

Television directors choose the angle of every camera shot, they determine the distance between the camera and every object being photographed,

How sound effects help you "see"

Sound effects are important because they work with the camera's pictures to convince you that what you see is really happening on your TV screen. In some shows, including one-hour dramas and made-for-TV movies, sound effects are added after filming. These effects are created by people called "foley artists," who get their name from Jack Foley, the Hollywood sound man who first developed the idea of adding sounds after filming. Can you match up each sound listed below in the left column with the way a foley artist would make it (see right column)? Then check your answers on page 95.

Sound You Hear	How the Sound Is Made
1. rain falling	**a.** squeezing a closed box of corn starch
2. gun being taken out of a holster	**b.** snapping carrots and celery into pieces
3. footsteps crunching in snow	**c.** punching a supermarket chicken
4. bones cracking	**d.** crinkling cellophane
5. egg frying	**e.** rubbing a doorknob against leather
6. hitting and punching noises	**f.** pouring bird seed over a ping pong ball

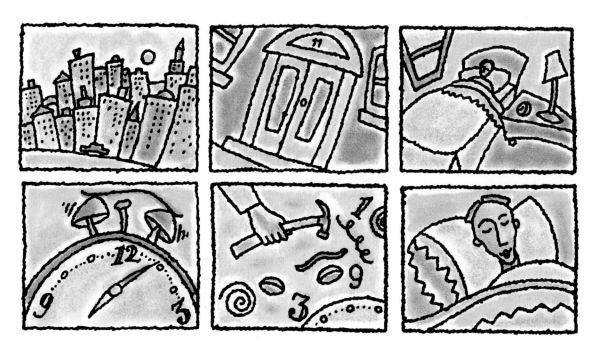

and they decide how long you will see each shot on your TV screen. They make these decisions long before the actual shooting of a show takes place and they record them on a storyboard, a kind of detailed comic strip of the entire show. The storyboard sets out what kinds of pictures and sounds are required, shot by shot, so that everyone on the production crew (the people who design the sets, the costumes, and select the lighting) knows just what the directors have in mind.

Get the Right Angle

Directors have lots of choices when it comes to picking the angle the camera will shoot from. A high-angle shot makes whatever's being photographed look small or less important because it is shot from above. This shot gives you, the viewer, a feeling of power because you seem larger than what you're looking at. High-angle shots can also show you something that the characters can't see and, for this reason, are used to build suspense on detective shows and mysteries. When you see the detective in the deserted warehouse far below, moving unknowingly straight towards the crooks, you know that he's headed for trouble before he does.

The opposite kind of shot, a low-angle shot, is taken from below an object and looks up at it. It makes whatever's being photographed look larger or more important than the viewer. For instance, a low-angle shot of a skyscraper taken at knee-level emphasizes how tall the building is and how short you are by comparison. Depending on the circumstances, a low-angle shot can make you chuckle or fill you with fear. Imagine lying on your back and opening your eyes to find a Saint Bernard dog licking your face. It might be funny if the dog is your pet – or scary if it isn't!

A "normal" or eye-level shot is used most of the time, in most TV shows. It's the same angle at which people usually look at each other and so it's a familiar, comfortable angle for viewing things. Unlike high-angle and low-angle shots, an eye-level shot doesn't "comment" at all on what's being photographed.

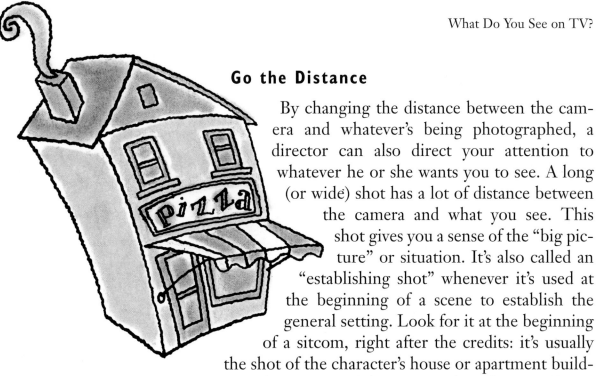

Go the Distance

By changing the distance between the camera and whatever's being photographed, a director can also direct your attention to whatever he or she wants you to see. A long (or wide) shot has a lot of distance between the camera and what you see. This shot gives you a sense of the "big picture" or situation. It's also called an "establishing shot" whenever it's used at the beginning of a scene to establish the general setting. Look for it at the beginning of a sitcom, right after the credits: it's usually the shot of the character's house or apartment building where most of the action takes place. Different

The lowdown on laugh tracks

The pre-recorded sound of audience laughter is called the laugh track. Does hearing a laugh track as you're watching your favourite sitcom help make you laugh? Maybe – but that's not the only reason why it's there. A laugh track gives you time to "get" the joke you've just heard. Without it, the characters would keep talking and you would be too busy listening to laugh. A laugh track also fills in any awkward silences when nothing interesting is going on in the sitcom. Cartoons and dramas use background music during those moments but comedy shows, which don't have background music, use laughter instead. Even shows that are taped in front of a live audience sometimes use recorded laughter. If the studio laughter isn't loud enough or hearty enough, the sound editors ask the audience to laugh on cue while they record some extra chuckles, chortles, and guffaws. During editing, these sounds are added to the original laughter to beef it up and make it even better!

kinds of shows have different establishing shots. On a talk show, for instance, this shot might include the whole stage and the audience.

A medium shot has less distance between the camera and an object than a wide shot. In this kind of shot, the person or object you're looking at is just as important as what's behind them. (You will usually see a person from the chest up.) Most shots on TV are medium shots.

A close-up shot moves in very close and directs your attention to an object or person, or a specific part of them. Look for close-up shots on talk shows and soap operas, especially when the actors or talk show guests are talking about a highly emotional topic. Directors rely on a lot of close-ups to keep you so involved with the people on TV that you'll continue to watch their program. Another kind of close-up shot, the extreme close-up, isn't used very often on TV. If you do see this kind of shot, it will probably be in a scary movie. Seeing a huge eyeball right up close, for example, can really startle and shock you!

Now Comes the Hard Part!

After taping and during editing, the director makes the final decision about which camera shots will be used in the show. And there can be lots of shots to choose from! Most sitcoms, for example, are taped twice in front of an audience and then twice without an audience. Three or four cameras, each at a different angle and distance, are used each time as the scenes are shot out of sequence. After taping, the very best shots are selected and pieced together in the correct order, a process that can take up to 50 hours for a single half-hour episode.

Time for a Change

How long will the viewer see each shot? That must also be decided during the editing of the show. Part of the tension in suspenseful shows and dramas is created by short shots and quick cuts, or camera changes. Getting viewers to pay attention when there are lots of changes can backfire, however. If the cuts come too fast, things on the TV screen look almost blurry and viewers stop following what's going on. You may have noticed this in some commercials or music videos, two places where this technique is used all the time.

Eye-Catching Effects

A lot of special camera effects are also created during editing. Slowing down or speeding up the tape creates slow and fast motion. An actor can be made to

TV tidbit

After a TV show has been shot and edited, any problems with the dialogue are corrected and music and sound effects are added. Directors refer to this as "sweetening."

Seeing is believing

If you could take a long, close-up look at some of the things you see on TV, you would discover that they aren't what they appear to be. Food is often made of rubber because it lasts longer under the hot lights during taping. A rubber roasted ham looks fake up close but if it's sprayed with glycerine (a clear, sticky liquid) to make it appear moist, shot from a distance, and shown to you for no more than 30 seconds, you'll probably think it's good enough to eat!

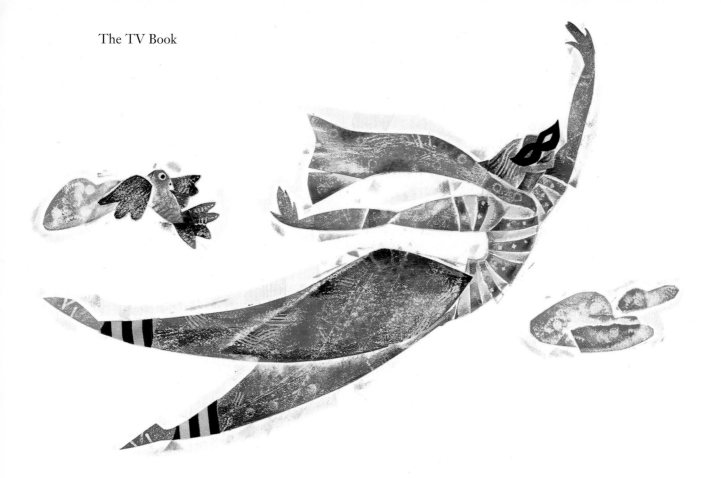

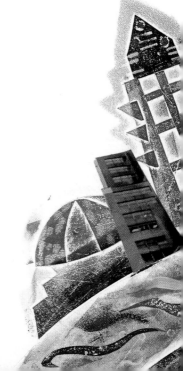

disappear by simply cutting out the piece of tape where he steps away from the camera's view. And joining together three different shots can create the illusion that a superhero has jumped off the ground and landed on top of a tall building. For this particular effect, the first shot would show the super hero crouched down, preparing to leap. The second shot would reveal her leaping through the air, thanks to an off-camera trampoline that she is bouncing on, and the third shot would show her landing on a roof. As you watch this sequence, you mentally "fill in the blanks" between each shot, allowing yourself to believe in the events you've been shown.

Directors use other camera effects to help you focus on the important things, react to them, and quickly fill in the missing pieces. Flashbacks, those moments when a TV character recalls something that happened much earlier, are often indicated by black-and-white shots, instead of colour ones. A jiggly hand-held camera effect that looks like a home-made video gives you the impression that whatever's being taped is happening right at that moment, without a TV director's help. Some shows use this "you-are-there" camera technique to make crime re-enactments performed by actors seem more real. However, a hand-held effect can also make some viewers think that what they're watching is really happening, or has really happened, and this isn't always true.

Now that you know more about what you see on your TV, you'll probably spot camera angles, effects, and other techniques that you've never noticed before. Why are the directors using a certain camera effect? How do you react when you see the effect? What else is going on and should you accept everything you see at first glance? Finding out the answers to these questions is part of the fun of being a tuned-in TV watcher and really seeing what's on TV!

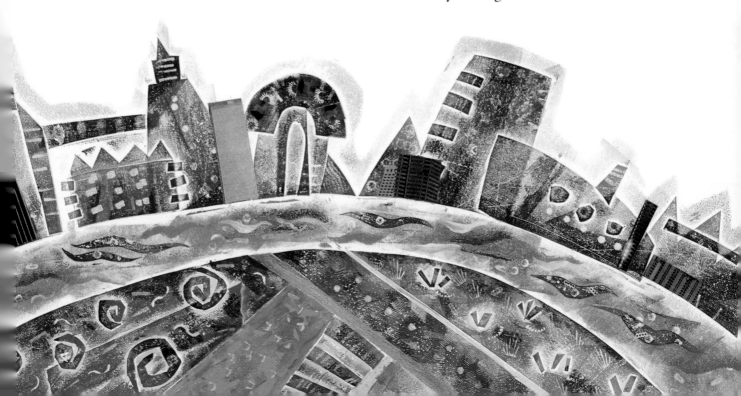

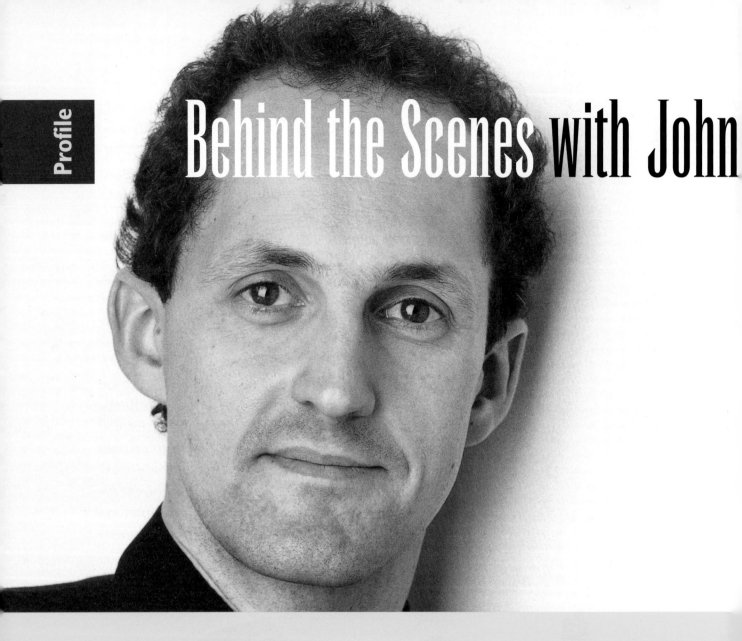

Behind the Scenes with John

Meet John Nelles – he's a TV actor and stunt person. John also teaches fight skills to other actors and specializes in sword fighting and hand-to-hand combat on the stage. During his career, John has played everything from miners to lawyers, done the voices for animated cartoon shows, and been "shot" and "wounded" many times!

Nelles

Interviewer: How do actors and stunt people make fights look so real on TV?

John: A lot of what you see on TV has to do with where the camera is. A camera sees height and width but it doesn't see depth. Let's say that I'm standing about three feet in front of you and the camera is looking over my shoulder. If I swing my arm as though I'm going to hit you in the face and your head snaps back, it will appear as though I've really hit you, even though I'm not close enough to touch you. Later the foley artist adds the sound effects. That also helps to trick you into thinking the punch really happened. It takes many experts working together to make the effect look exciting and appear real – it's definitely not something people should try to copy at home.

Interviewer: What about sword fighting – how do you make that look real?

John: Some actors haven't had training to do sword fights. When I'm hired as the fight choreographer, it's my job to show them the moves and make them look like experts. Sometimes I only teach them what they have to know. They use the same move over and over and it's just shot from different angles, using close-ups to make it even more exciting. When you put all of the shots together and add sound effects and music, it looks like a big fight.

Interviewer: So cameras do a lot of the work?

John: That's right. The other important thing to remember is that the viewers want to believe what

49

they're seeing. They want to believe that the hero is fighting the other person. However, the moment that the viewers believe that the actor is actually getting hurt, they stop believing the story and the characters, and they only worry about the actor. Knowing that the stunts are done safely allows us to let our imaginations go, and enjoy the TV show.

Interviewer: Do actors use real guns on TV?

John: The bottom line in all of this work is safety. There are very, very strict rules about who can handle guns on a set. An actor uses a gun that can safely shoot blanks when their character has to actually fire the gun. The minute the scene is over, the weapons handler comes over and takes the gun away. The rest of the time, you usually use a fake made of rubber, or a replica of the real gun, that can't fire.

Interviewer: Doesn't a rubber gun look fake?

John: No, fake guns look very real, even up close. Fake blood looks real, too. It's often corn syrup with food colouring. There's even fake glass that's used when someone is thrown through a window or has a bottle smashed on their head. It's called "breakaway glass" or "candy glass" and it's made of sugar.

Interviewer: Are computers changing the way stunts are done these days?

John: Computer-generated special effects can help make exciting-looking stunts even more exciting. I played a soldier in a war movie and computers were used to generate most of the landing craft that carried the soldiers. We had only two real landing craft, but the computers made it look like there were 50 of them coming in together.

Interviewer: Some people say that TV violence is bad to watch because it doesn't show the real consequences of violence. What do you think?

John: Violence is a very real part of our world and I don't think that it does any good to pretend that it doesn't exist. But I think it's important not to show violence just for the sake of making something more exciting. That's what I don't like about the Mighty Morphin Power Rangers and Teenage Mutant Ninja Turtles – they solve all their problems by using violence right away. As soon as they see an enemy, they fight. Kids like these shows because they're exciting and it makes them feel powerful, but they need to understand that these actors are fighting in a safe way and, in their lives, it's better to solve a problem by talking about it.

Interviewer: Have you ever hurt yourself while fighting?

John: Once, when I was teaching fighting, I broke one of my fingers. I was telling someone, "Make sure you don't do this!" as I demonstrated a move, and just by chance one of my fingers caught a piece of cloth and bent the wrong way. Some stunt people get hurt from time to time, although it doesn't happen very often because they're very, very careful about fighting and other stunts. A stunt person knows that it takes lots of training to throw a punch without breaking your wrist – or hurting anyone else.

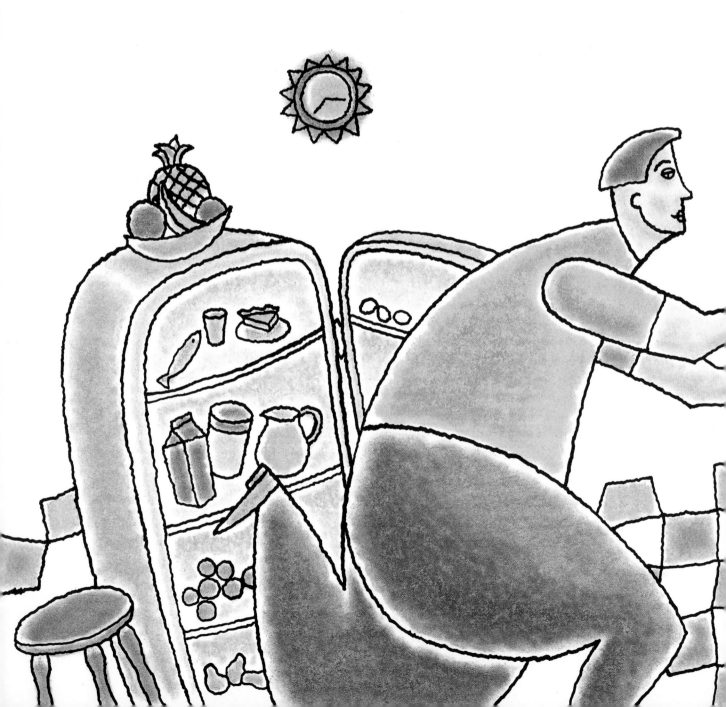

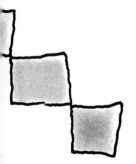

You're watching your favourite show, it's just getting to a really good part and then . . . a commercial. What do you do? Go to the kitchen? Press the mute button? Watch the commercial?

If you're an average TV viewer, you'll find yourself in this situation many, many times – during a year, you see (or perhaps choose not to see) at least 20,000 commercials. Commercials pay for most of the programs you watch: networks charge advertisers to air the advertisers' ads, then use the money they receive to cover the costs of producing the shows. But TV advertising isn't limited to just commercials. There are other kinds of ads on TV as well.

These Things Just "Ad" Up!

Sometimes you watch an ad on TV without even knowing that's what it is. A well-known soft drink prominently displayed during a prime-time TV show, a Saturday morning cartoon with popular characters that are also toys you can buy, "infomercials," and even music videos are, in fact, advertisements. They're all intended to persuade you to buy something, whether it's a can of cola, an action toy, an amazing new mop, or a compact disc.

How effective are these kinds of ads at convincing you to buy their products? When MTV, an American music video channel, started showing videos in 1981, music sales boomed. Record companies found that actually being able to see bands perform their songs made people more likely to buy the group's records and concert tickets. If you've ever watched MuchMusic, Canada's music video station, or MTV you know how hard it is to stop watching videos. The constantly changing camera shots, unusual camera angles and, of course, memorable music are exactly the same things advertisers use in "regular" commercials to get your attention and make sure you remember their ad.

Some TV Tricks of the Trade

Advertisers use other techniques, as well, to get your attention and hold it for the entire length of a commercial. Here are just some of those techniques:

• Repeating the ad over and over again. Studies

What's an "infomercial"?

An infomercial is a commercial as long as a TV program that claims to give you information (or "info") about the product being advertised. Unlike ordinary commercials, infomercials often look like talk shows with a studio audience and famous people as guests or hosts. These singers, actors, and athletes help advertise the product in the infomercial by talking about it and trying it out. In 1994, infomercials sold about one billion American dollars' worth of products in the U.S., including everything from psychic hotlines to spray-on hair. Infomercials have become a popular way to advertise because they don't cost as much to make and air as other TV ads. They usually appear on TV during Saturday afternoons or the middle of the night, when ad rates are lowest. And for the same money it takes to make two half-minute commercials, advertisers can make one 30-minute infomercial. Infomercials even have their own commercial breaks, which interrupt the main part of the infomercial to urge you to buy the product right away. ("Call this toll-free number to place your order now!") That's right – commercials *within* commercials!

show that, if you have a choice, many people are more likely to buy an advertised brand instead of an unadvertised brand, even an unadvertised brand that's cheaper. One reason you're familiar with the advertised brand name is that you've heard the ad for it over and over again.

- Using camera effects and special effects. Close-ups can make products look larger than they are. Computer-generated special effects can make toys appear to do something, such as move by themselves, that they won't actually do when you get them home.
- Emphasizing "premiums," the toys or prizes that

come with certain products. The "special gift inside" may be the only reason you buy the cereal.

- Showing or saying words such as "free," "new," "amazing," and "improved" to get everyone's attention. (Did someone say "free"?)
- Hiring famous people to tell you to buy a certain product. Advertisers conduct surveys to find out which celebrities you trust and like the most, then use those people to promote their products.

There are limits, however, to the extent advertisers can use these techniques to convince you to buy their products. Your government – the Canadian Radio-Television and Telecommunications Commission (CRTC) in Canada and the Federal Communications Commission (FCC) in the U.S. – has hundreds of rules to guarantee that the television industry serves you and the "public interest." As a Canadian or American citizen, you literally own the airwaves that the TV networks use for broadcasting. The networks are allowed to "borrow" the airwaves provided that what they broadcast meets the needs of the public.

TV tidbit

Advertisers often spend more creating a commercial that lasts one minute than TV producers spend making a half-hour show. Between 20 and 40 percent of a product's price goes to pay for the cost of advertising it, including its commercials. So if you buy a toy that costs $29.95, between $6 and $12 of your money goes to telling you and others about it!

They Don't Kid Around with Kids!

The networks, governments, and advertisers agree that children are a special part of the TV audience. Kids under five years of age don't understand that commercials are there to sell them something. (To

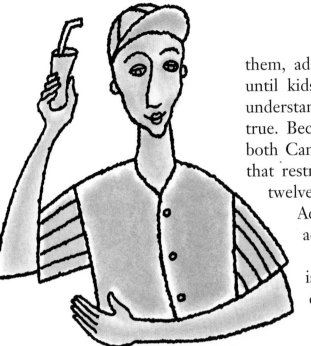

them, ads are just shorter programs.) And it isn't until kids are about eight years of age that they understand that commercials aren't always literally true. Because of this, the advertising industries in both Canada and the U.S. must obey special rules that restrict what can be advertised to kids under twelve and how it can be advertised to them.

According to the rules, advertisers can't take advantage of you by having a baseball player tell you how great a particular brand of bat is, for example. He can endorse a sports drink, but not a bat or a baseball. What's the difference? Bats and baseballs are too close-

Take a break!

Slogans are those snappy, memorable lines that help you remember a product's name. The ones below have each appeared in a real TV commercial. See if you can match up each slogan in the left column with the product it advertises in the right column. Then check your answers on page 95. Do the slogans make sense when you see them removed from the music, special effects, and fast cuts that are part of their commercials?

1. there's nothing more powerful under the sun

2. doing it right

3. taste beyond belief

4. something right to grow up on

5. the best a man can get

6. it just feels right

7. the ultimate in care

a. diapers

b. peanut butter

c. a car

d. shaving gel

e. cheese slices

f. a department store

g. dish soap

57

ly identified with what the player does for a living. Seeing him advertise either a bat or a baseball could leave you with the impression that you'll play like him if you buy one, too. Computer-generated effects in commercials are okay, as long as there's at least one part of the ad that shows the product as it actually is. If a toy plane can't fly on its own, the ad has

Do some ads make you mad?

When you see a TV ad that you think is misleading or untrue, take action! If you live in Canada, write to the Advertising Standards Council of Advertising Standards Canada. You can also write to CBC's *Street Cents*, a consumer-oriented TV show for kids and teenagers. If you live in the U.S., write to the Children's Advertising Review Unit of the Council of Better Business Bureaus, the Federal Trade Commission, and your state Attorney General. You can also write to a magazine for kids, called *Zillions*, and tell them about it: *Zillions* is published by the Consumers Union, a nonprofit organization that aims to give consumers the information they need to spend their money wisely. And, whether you live in Canada or the U.S., you can always write to the network on whose station an ad appeared. You'll find the addresses for all of these organizations on pages 93-5. (If you see the ad on a local, independent station or on a cable station, you'll need to contact the station and get their address. Then, write to the general manager or the person who handles complaints.) You can also write to the company whose product is advertised and to the celebrity who appears in the ad, if the ad has one. Your local library has reference books listing advertisers' addresses and the addresses for actors' agents, the people who usually receive the actors' mail: ask the librarian for help finding what you need. When you do complain about a TV ad, be specific. Include the name of the product, the problem with it, the show and station that the ad appeared on, and the time of day when you saw it.

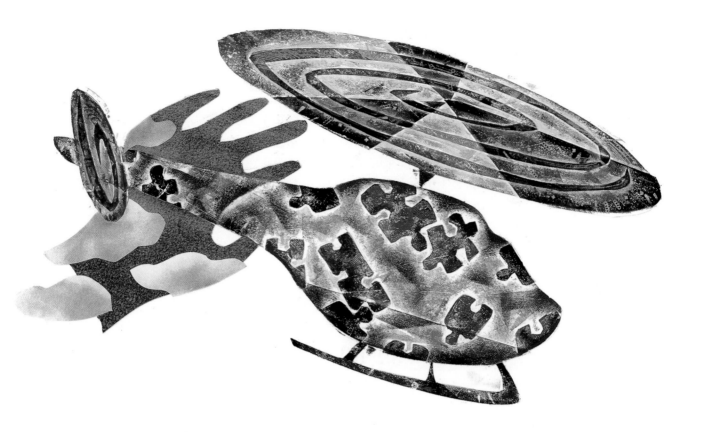

to show someone's hand holding the plane.

Two U.S. toy companies had to pay large fines when the Federal Trade Commission (the government department that investigates citizens' complaints about TV commercials) decided that their ads were misleading people. In one ad, a toy helicopter was made to look as if it could actually fly when it couldn't, and in another ad a ballerina doll was made to look like it could stand and twirl all by itself without being held. Other toy companies have been fined for showing two toys together without clearly stating that they were sold separately and for showing a toy in one piece when it actually came in several pieces.

There are many organizations watching out for

you to make sure that advertisers aren't "stretching the truth" to persuade you to buy their products. (You'll find a list of organizations concerned with kids and TV advertising listed in the back of this book, along with information about what they do.) Some of these organizations are consumer "watch-dog" groups that monitor TV ads to make sure they're telling the truth. One American watchdog group is The Center for Science in the Public Interest.

Batteries not included

Advertisers are required to show or say "disclaimers," such as "batteries not included," in toy and cereal ads. Here's your chance to find out what advertisers are really saying when they use these phrases. Find the disclaimer in the left column, then look directly beside it, in the right column, for its meaning.

The Disclaimer Says:	What the Disclaimer Really Means:
"Some assembly required"	You have to put the toy together before it will work
"Accessories sold separately"	All the great stuff you see in this commercial doesn't come with this toy
"Batteries not included"	You must buy batteries and put them in the toy before it will work
"Part of a complete breakfast"	If you eat this cereal with certain nutritious foods such as milk, fruit, and toast, then you will have a completely nutritious breakfast

Every year, they give away the Harlan Page Hubbard Memorial Awards – fake-gold trophies topped with real lemons – to advertisers with the most misleading advertisements.

Calling All Shoppers!

Why do advertisers bother trying to reach kids when there are so many restrictions on what advertisers can say and do on TV? Because kids are a very important, very profitable market. In Canada, *TG Magazine,* a teen publication, estimates that Canadian teenagers spend a total of more than eighty million dollars (Canadian) a week. According to the Children's Advertising Review Unit, American parents give their children approximately six billion dollars (American) each year in allowances.

As well as spending your own money, you influence what your family buys. And even if you don't have any money to spend now, you will in a few years. You are the customers of tomorrow and any advertising that builds "brand loyalty" (your loyalty or faithfulness to a particular brand or product) will pay off in the years ahead.

Coming Your Way – More TV Ads!

To reach kids like you, advertisers are finding new places where they can advertise their products. American businessman Chris Whittle started *Channel One News,* a 12-minute newscast beamed daily into 10,000 schools across the U.S. that also carries advertising. Schools that subscribe to the

61

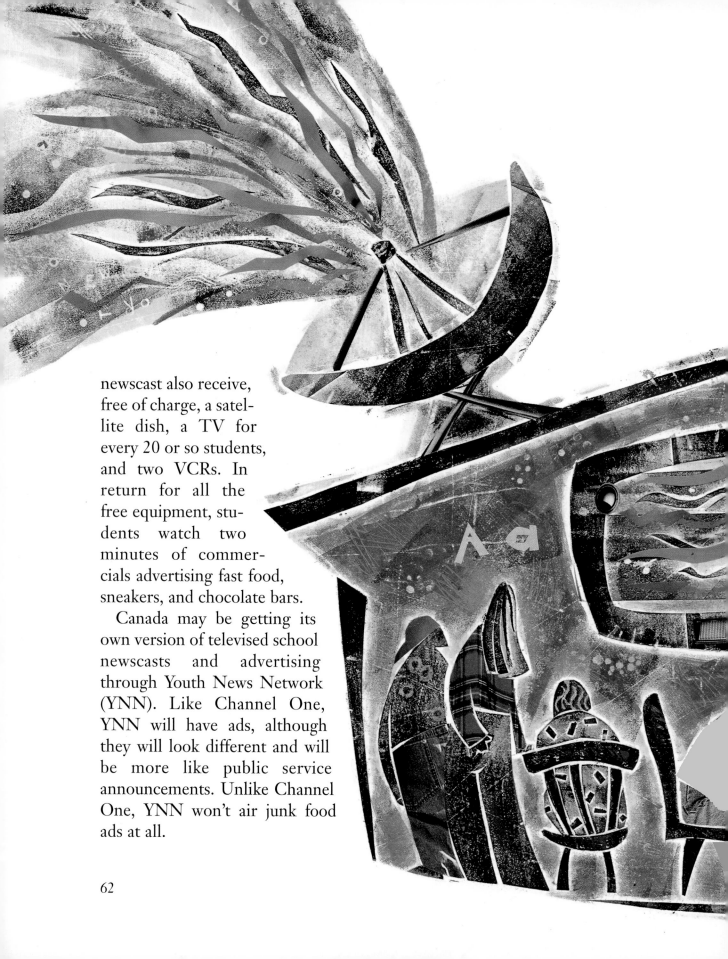

newscast also receive, free of charge, a satellite dish, a TV for every 20 or so students, and two VCRs. In return for all the free equipment, students watch two minutes of commercials advertising fast food, sneakers, and chocolate bars.

Canada may be getting its own version of televised school newscasts and advertising through Youth News Network (YNN). Like Channel One, YNN will have ads, although they will look different and will be more like public service announcements. Unlike Channel One, YNN won't air junk food ads at all.

Do TV commercials have a place in your classroom? A lot of people think they don't. They believe that businesses shouldn't be able to choose which messages, through news stories and advertising, are heard in classrooms. They also believe that businesses shouldn't be able to make a profit from students who are forced to watch the TV newscast in their classrooms each day. There are also plenty of commercial-free news programs available for broadcast in schools.

Other people disagree. They believe that the advantages of having the free equipment and receiving the newscasts outweigh the disadvantages.

Whether you watch TV advertising while you're at school or at home, it's up to you to think about the ads you see and make up your own mind about what to buy and why you should buy it. After all, advertisers know that there are many reasons you buy a product – and only one of those reasons is because you need it.

Behind the Scenes with Rebecca

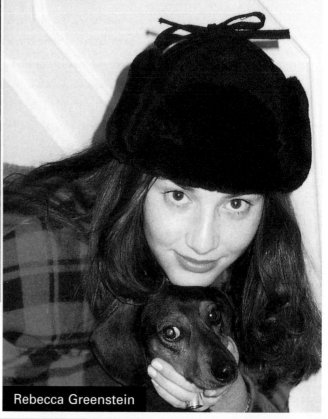

Dalia Rotstein

Rebecca Greenstein

When Rebecca and Dalia were twelve years old, they came up with an unusual idea for a science project. They decided to find out about TV advertising by looking at the scientific experiments in some TV commercials. With their amazing project, Rebecca and Dalia became winners at their school's science fair – and went on to compete at the annual Canada-Wide Science Fair!

Greenstein and Dalia Rotstein

Interviewer: What was the main idea behind your science fair project?

Dalia: The purpose was to look at brand-name products which have scientific experiments presented in TV ads. We looked at the commercials for several of these products, then we did the experiments ourselves to see how well they worked outside the commercial. As well, we took some of each product's competitors and tested them in the same experiments.

Rebecca: We also made up our own variations of the TV experiments and tried those too. We did that to extend our knowledge and make our project a more unique science project that it would have been if we had just done what we saw on TV.

Interviewer: Why did you decide to look at advertising for your project?

Rebecca: Commercials are something we're exposed to every day and we take them at face value. Kids, especially, are always taught to see things and not really question them. Basically, we wanted to do the experiments we saw on TV and see how well they worked in real life. That's the main idea behind most science projects: you notice something that you see every day, you get curious about it, and you wonder why it is that way.

Interviewer: Were you surprised at the results you got?

Rebecca: We didn't expect any of our results to be wildly different from what was shown on TV. But at the same time, we didn't expect them to turn out exactly the same way.

Dalia: We tried the experiments for five different products. One product worked perfectly and two didn't work at all the way they did on TV. The other two products were somewhere in between.

Interviewer: Did you contact the companies whose products you tested?

Dalia: Yes, we did, at the beginning of our project. A lot of the companies sent stuff to us describing their experiments, including instructions for doing the experiments. It was very interesting to receive their results. Some companies also sent instructions for other experiments, not just the TV ones. Some of the companies were more willing to do this than others and one company said they couldn't send us anything because their stuff was confidential.

Rebecca: After we finished our project, we wrote to the companies again. We just told them we would be sharing our results at the Canada-Wide Science Fair. We told them that if they had any comments or questions on how we conducted our experiments, please feel free to contact us. That was a long time ago. I hope eventually we'll get a response, but it's hard to say.

Interviewer: How did you find the names of the companies and their addresses?

Rebecca: We looked on the products' packages. Sometimes they give mailing addresses right on the box. That's how we got a lot of our mailing information.

Interviewer: Now that you've done a science project on TV advertising, what do you think of TV advertising in general?

Dalia: I think a lot of advertising is unclear and takes advantage of the fact that you're not really paying close attention because it's only a commercial.

Rebecca: I think people should look at TV advertising a lot more critically and question everything they see and are told. You really have to go and find out yourself.

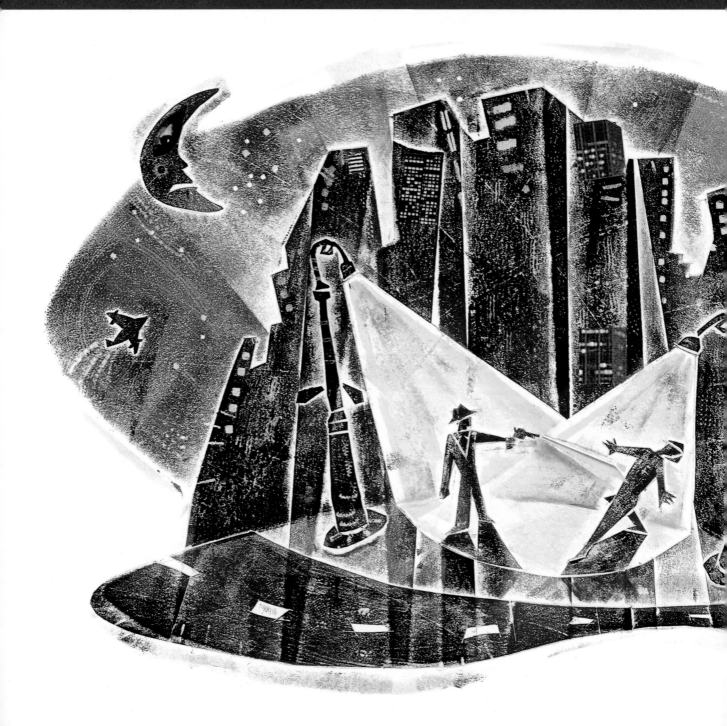

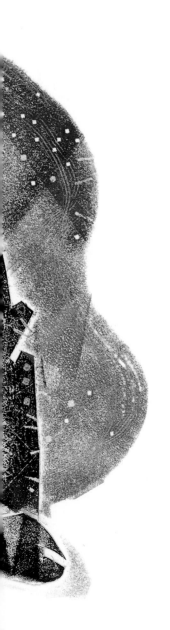

s, Blood and Gore

You're flipping through the channels, and there is nothing good on TV. Everything looks boring, until...POW! Some guy just got punched in the stomach. What's happening here? Before you know it, you're watching two guys duking it out over some unknown "disagreement." If this scene seems familiar, you won't be surprised to hear that you will likely see about 8,000 murders and 100,000 other violent acts on TV – all before you graduate from elementary school!

Why is there so much violence on TV? The people who make TV shows use fights, shootings, and other kinds of violent acts to hold your attention and keep you from channel surfing. They know that it's more exciting to watch two characters resolve a problem in a shootout than it is to see the same characters discussing their differences politely. Sudden violent events also quickly take care of any problems that are part of the show's plot – killing the "bad guys," for instance, is a handy way to get rid of them by the end of the show.

What's the Big Deal, Anyway?

Most researchers believe that watching violence on TV makes TV viewers, especially kids, act more violently in their own lives. Many studies show that, after you watch a violent program, you are more likely to imitate what you've just seen on TV – shoving and checking like a hockey star, kicking like a Power Ranger, or wrestling like your hero on the *World Wrestling Federation*. Watching people you admire and respect behaving in violent ways makes it seem all right for you to copy their behaviour.

A small number of studies have found that watching violent TV programs doesn't mean you'll automatically grow up to be a violent adult. But many studies – and there have been 3,000 studies since the 1950s! – agree on one thing: heavy watchers of violent TV are more aggressive than light viewers.

More Bad News about TV Violence

Many experts caution that watching violence affects you in more ways than just making you aggressive. It's been proven that people who watch a lot of violent TV are slower to offer help to victims than people who didn't watch violent TV, because they're not as bothered by the pain and suffering of real victims. Maybe you've

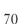

noticed that it's easier to watch your favourite horror movie for the fourth time than it was the first time. The more you see something, the less it shocks and scares you.

How do you complain about a too-violent TV show?

In both Canada and the U.S., write first to the general manager or president of the TV station on which the show appeared, being sure to state the name of the program and the time and date it appeared. Send the letter immediately after you see the program. The station's review committee will watch the show, then write you personally within several weeks of receiving your letter. In Canada, if you're not satisfied with the station's response, write or e-mail the Canadian Broadcast Standards Council (CBSC) within two weeks of getting the station's letter. The CBSC will meet to decide whether the station has broken the anti-violence code, and you'll receive notice of their decision. (Be patient; it may take a while to receive a response.) If the CBSC decides that the station has broken the code, the station must broadcast a statement during prime-time, within 30 days, saying that it has broken the code, and the offending show cannot be shown again. In the United States, if you're not satisfied with the station's response, you can write to the Federal Communications Commission (FCC). Be sure to include your full name and address, the name and city of the station, the name of the program, the time and date it appeared, and an account of what the local station did do in response to your complaint. The FCC can file your complaint against the TV station and consider it when the station's licence is due for renewal (every seven years). For addresses and more info about organizations that you can contact about TV violence, see pages 93-5.

71

TV programs don't usually show the real consequences, or effects, of violence, so it's easy for you to assume that punches don't hurt and bullets don't kill. (If punches don't appear to hurt, you may be more likely to punch, too.) Instead of spending weeks in a coma followed by months of recovery, a TV victim is cured and back in time for next week's show. TV fights go on much longer than real fights would; in real life one punch to someone's face would tend to break the puncher's hand and knock the victim unconscious.

You be the judge!

At one time or another, each of the following have been considered violent acts. Which ones do you think are violent?

• the Three Stooges poking each other in the eye ☐ violent ☐ not violent

• scenes of war on the 6:00 news ☐ violent ☐ not violent

• a food fight ☐ violent ☐ not violent

• someone being threatened with a gun ☐ violent ☐ not violent

• a nasty insult ☐ violent ☐ not violent

• a cartoon character shooting another character ☐ violent ☐ not violent

Clowning Around on Kids' Cartoons

Some people who study TV violence think that kids' cartoons are the most violent programs on television. Why? After Elmer Fudd shoots Bugs Bunny, Bugs shows up as good as new in the next scene. Television viewers don't see the real-life effects of a violent act. Violence in cartoons can make you believe that killing or hurting others is funny.

Who Knows What to Do?

Television violence is a complicated issue, and that's why it's taken so long for governments, experts on TV violence, and the TV industry to decide what to do about it. No one, including the many groups concerned about TV violence (see pages 93-5), can seem to agree on the best way to protect you while not taking away anyone else's right to free speech and creative freedom. Some people think that stations and networks should be fined if they don't

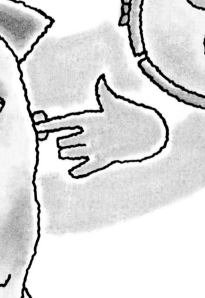

reduce violent programming and increase non-violent programming. Others think that warnings should appear on your TV screen before violent shows, announcing that violence is bad for your health.

Who's Got the Control?

The CRTC (the Canadian broadcasting authority) decided, after much debate, to limit the rights of Canadian adults to see anything they want in order to protect Canadian kids (the new violence code, like the advertising regulations, seeks to protect kids under twelve). The government encouraged Canadian broadcasters to come up with a code, or set of rules, that they will voluntarily follow. Broadcasters must follow the code or their licence to broadcast may not be renewed. They've agreed to show very little violence in kids' programs, and the little that there is has to be essential to the story. (Turn to page 90 to read more about the Canadian code.)

The U.S. government said that the American television industry had to cut back on the number of violent shows or they'd pass a law that would force them to reduce TV violence. Although many people who work in TV – producers, network executives, actors – felt the government was interfering with their right to freedom of speech, in 1992 three U.S. networks (ABC, CBS, and NBC) issued a statement outlining what steps they were prepared to take to limit TV violence (see page 92).

TV tidbit

In December, 1994 a newspaper in Bombay, India reported that hundreds of high-rise apartment dwellers threw their TVs out their windows to protest against violence and sex on Indian television – now that's something you shouldn't try at home!

How old should you be to watch violent TV shows?

The makers of TV shows follow guidelines that protect kids under twelve from too much TV violence. These guidelines are based on research gathered by experts who have studied children. According to the experts, a child can't tell the difference between real and make-believe until they're around five years old. By the time a kid is eight years old, however, they no longer believe everything they see and hear. If you were in charge of deciding what a kid could watch on TV, what would you do if:

1. A newscast with pictures of a real person being shot was on TV?
   I would let the kid watch it if they were:
   a) five years old   **b)** eight years old   **c)** twelve years old **d)** any age

2. A horror movie was on TV?
   I would let the kid watch it if they were:
   a) five years old   **b)** eight years old   **c)** twelve years old **d)** any age

3. A show that features a group of high-kicking superheroes who fight evil monsters was on TV?
   I would let the kid watch it if they were:
   a) five years old   **b)** eight years old   **c)** twelve years old **d)** any age

4. A cartoon, starring a character who tries to capture and eat another character despite repeatedly blowing himself up and being injured, was on TV?
   I would let the kid watch it if they were:
   a) five years old   **b)** eight years old   **c)** twelve years old **d)** any age

Some TV stations in the U.S. are taking action by reducing violence on the news. "Family-sensitive" newscasts, which began in Minneapolis on WCCO-TV, have spread to other local stations across the

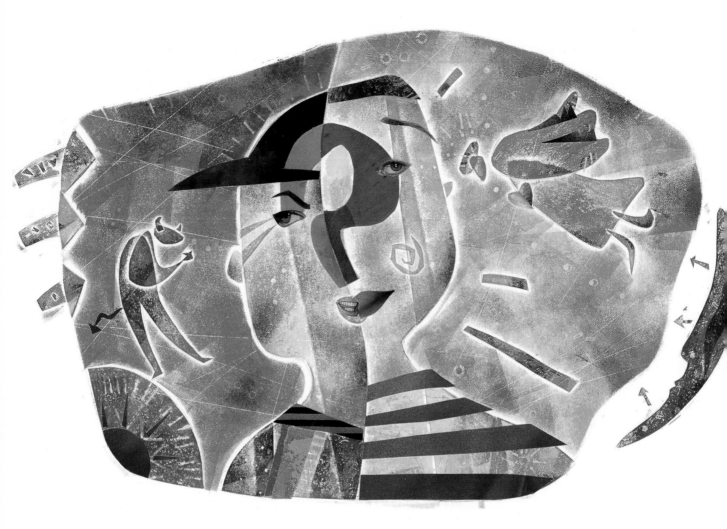

U.S. Instead of images of flashing ambulance lights and bloodstained pavement, these stations air more stories about issues that affect the community and show how citizens can become involved.

The Canadian and American governments may have found a way to give control over what kids watch to parents rather than governments or networks. In 1996, the CRTC decided that the makers of TV sets had to build in a device that will block out violent shows in Canada, and the U.S. Congress passed a Bill that made it law in the U.S. The device is called a V Chip, or viewer control chip, and was invented by an engineer at Simon Fraser University in British Columbia. With a V Chip, your parents can choose among kinds of violence you are allowed to see and each network will send out coded information before each program airs. So if a Real Crime show is coded higher than the ratings your parents set, it will be blocked out. The V Chip has been tested in homes across Canada and the United States. While the rating categories have now been adopted and are shown at the beginning of TV shows (except sports and news) on most North American TV networks, the V Chip is not yet widely available. TV sets built since Christmas 1998 will have built-in V Chips.

In Canada, the Canadian Association of Broadcasters (CAB) and the Canadian Cable Television Association (CCTA), and in the United States, the National Association of Broadcasters (NAB), developed their country's V Chip rating system. Although the names given to the codes are slightly different, the ratings are essentially the same. In Canada, the specific warning about coarse language, etc., is spoken, which is particularly useful for parents who happen to be out of the room, but still within earshot, at the beginning of a TV show.

Of course, if you think the violence is too much on a particular show, you can do more than change the channel or turn off the TV. Write letters to tell advertisers, networks, producers, actors and your government representatives that you're not watching and ask them what they're doing to reduce TV violence. (See "How do you complain about a too-violent TV show?" on page 71. For tips on writing effective letters, see page 95.)

And when you do watch TV, keep an eye out for programs that show people who are being helpful, kind, and heroic. Why? Studies show that watching these shows may help you to be more like that, too!

Behind the Scene

Who took a stand against TV violence after her sister was murdered, organized a petition which over one million Canadians signed, and personally spoke to the Prime Minister about TV violence? Virginie Larivière did – and she was just thirteen years old at the time. As the result of her actions, the Canadian broadcasting industry introduced a voluntary code that limits TV violence.

with Virginie Larivière

Interviewer: What gave you the idea to start your petition?

Virginie: The violent death of my sister, Marie-Eve, changed everything for me. The rage and despair that I felt pushed me to act positively, instead of staying down in the dumps or sinking to crime and drugs. For me, creating this petition represented a concrete way of reducing violence in our society.

Interviewer: How did you start your petition?

Virginie: I spoke to my mother about it at Marie-Eve's funeral and then she mentioned it to my cousin, Diane. Diane liked my idea and asked if she could help me. I wrote my petition and we distributed it to all the schools in Quebec. Later, we contacted the media and I went on TV for the first time.

Interviewer: How did you go about collecting over one million signatures?

Virginie: Through TV, newspapers, and radio, people began to know me and agree with me. I travelled a great deal in Canada and I met as many people as possible. I worked very hard!

Interviewer: How did the government respond to your petition?

Virginie: The Prime Minister signed my petition, and after that, the television broadcasters created their own voluntary code of ethics, which the Canadian Radio-Television and Telecommunications Commission approved.

Interviewer: Does the voluntary code go far enough in reducing TV violence?

Virginie: I don't think so. Even so, it is a step in the right direction.

Interviewer: How do you define "violence"?

Virginie: For me, violence is everything that ignores the limits of respect. To humiliate, to hit, to hurt – these all come from not respecting oneself and not respecting others. We need to educate people about violence.

Interviewer: Some people say that kids watching TV violence can't be the only cause of violence in real life. It has to be the result of a lot of things, like poverty and easy access to weapons. What do you think?

Virginie: Violence is a complex thing whether it is real or invented. Violence in real life seems more serious because we see the consequences immediately. But when a child watches violence on TV, the consequences seem less serious because they don't show up until much later.

Interviewer: Do you think that cartoons should be removed from TV?

Virginie: Not all of them, but most of them, yes. Ninja Turtles, Power Rangers, and even Bugs Bunny should be removed. The heroes fight and hit each other and it isn't real. One cannot survive a fall off a cliff or an explosion from a bomb you are holding in your hands.

Interviewer: Do you think television makes people violent?

Virginie: It is proven that violence shown on television makes people more aggressive. Violent or not, TV influences people, especially children.

Interviewer: Do you think your actions have made a difference?

Virginie: Yes! People are more aware of violence and the government has finally taken action.

Keith Spicer, chair of the CRTC, has gone on record as saying, "Ms. Larivière had a profound impact on our national conscience, and her crusade was enormously influential in pushing TV violence to the top of the national agenda."

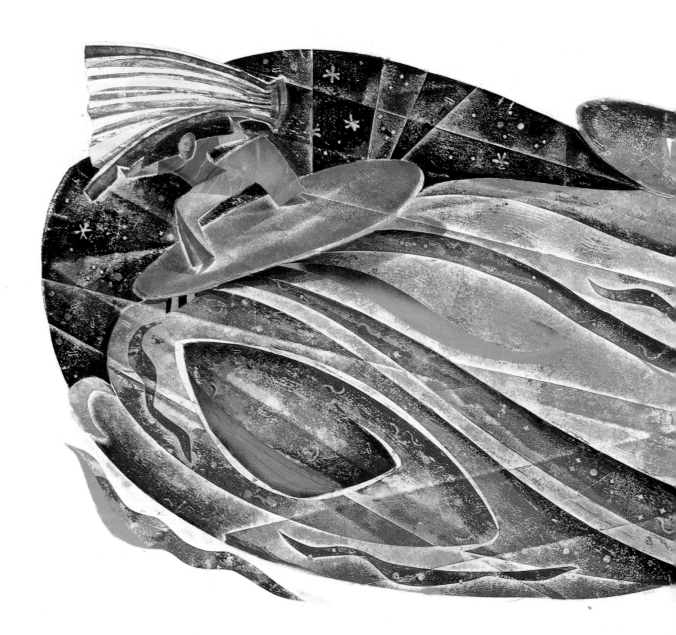

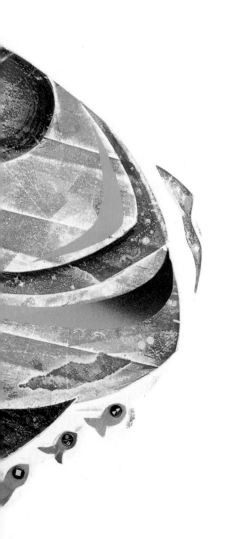

Imagine yourself in the year 2000, surfing your way through 500 channels. It could take hours to check out every TV channel. Think about the size of the TV guide!

Life with hundreds of TV channels – what some people call "the 500-channel universe" – isn't just a thing of the future. We're already on our way to increasing the number of channels available. Digital technology now makes it possible for signals from 10 TV channels to be compressed into a wire that used to carry one. A pizza-sized satellite dish that delivers about 150 channels is already on sale, and some cable companies predict they'll be offering 300 to 400 channels in the next few years.

Will you need to be a weightlifter just to pick up the TV guide for all these new channels? Probably not! If and when there are hundreds of channels, you'll likely use your remote control to browse through on-screen menus showing different program categories. As you select a category, more specific menus will appear, until you narrow down your choice to a particular program.

In a 500-channel universe, each channel – anything from all bowling to all soap operas – will appeal to a very specific audience, and TV commercials will probably look very different from the ones that you see today. Each channel's audience won't be as big as the audiences of today, but viewers will be more alike and, advertisers hope, more likely to buy their product. Because it costs less to buy advertising time on shows with smaller audiences, you'll probably see smaller companies (which have less money to spend on advertising) with commercials on TV. One day, you might see your own veterinarian advertising on the Chihuahua Channel!

A lot of people think that TV in the future won't be just for watching more programs or showing different kinds of commercials. You might use your TV set to play video games with your friend across town or choose books and magazines from a central "library" before reading them on your TV screen. Or perhaps you'll click a mouse on menus on your screen to order baseball tickets and pizza or use your TV set to see your friends while you talk to them on the phone. TV may be "interactive," which means that you may be able to actively participate in and respond to what you see and hear on your TV through the use of computers and other technology.

Nobody really knows exactly what the TV of the future will look like. However, everyone does agree that it will cost you money. Every time you use your interactive TV, you'll be charged for it. The charges will be sent to you in a TV bill that might look like today's phone bill.

Television in the future, just like television today, has the potential to affect your life in some important ways. What form it will take depends on you, your family and friends, and whether each of you uses it in new ways or not, and finds them helpful or not. What's on TV now, and in the future, depends on you, too. Write letters (by yourself or with your friends or your class), join organizations involved with TV (see "Back of the Book"), talk to your parents and friends and teachers about what you watch, question what you see, and talk back to your TV!

Tele-Wise Words

Here are some important words to do with television that you will find in this book.

Brand Loyalty: Loyalty or faithfulness to a particular brand or product name. TV commercials (and other forms of advertising) help develop brand loyalty in people by making them aware of a particular product's name, and encouraging them to buy the product because they are familiar with it.

Convention: Widely accepted feature of particular kinds of TV shows that viewers instantly recognize and understand. For instance, a convention of many TV sit-coms is the sound of audience laughter after an actor says something funny. Conventions are also used in other places, including the theatre.

Cut: Abrupt change from one shot to the other. Some TV commercials and music videos contain frequent cuts.

Director: The person who supervises the taping of a TV show. Among other things, a director chooses how the actors will act and which camera shots to use.

Dubbing: Adding a new soundtrack after the TV program has been shot. The new soundtrack may include a translation of the show's dialogue if the show airs on a foreign-language network.

Editing: Selecting the camera shots that will appear in a TV show and piecing them together in the order in which viewers will see them.

Endorse: To publicly approve of something or someone. Celebrities, well-known or famous people, often appear in TV commercials and infomercials to endorse particular products.

Focus Group: A group of people who are recruited to form a sample audience and who are asked to give their opinions about a particular TV show, especially a new one. This information is used by the show's makers to find out in advance what kind of people are likely to watch the show and what people like and don't like about it.

Foley Artist: The person who creates the sound effects which are added after a show has been shot. Foley artists are named after Jack Foley, the Hollywood sound man who first developed the idea of adding sounds after filming.

Infomercial: A commercial as long as a TV program that claims to give you information (or "info") about the product being advertised.

Interactive Television: In the not-so-distant future, you'll be able to use your television as a combination phone, computer, and television.

Licence: Paid-for permission to broadcast a TV show. A network must have a licence before it can air any programs.

Market: A group of people who might watch a certain TV show or buy a particular product.

Network: A group of television stations that are connected and which air the same TV shows and commercials.

Pilot: The first trial episode of a new show.

Prime-time: The time of the day during which the most people watch TV. Prime-time is from 8 to 11 p.m. Monday through Saturday, and 7 to 11 p.m. on Sunday.

Producer: The person who creates a TV show. A producer takes care of the business details and hires and supervises the people who do the creative work on the show, including the director and the scriptwriters.

Public Interest: What is considered to be best for people in general. In return for free use of the public airwaves, a network or independent station must serve the public interest, or the public good, usually by broadcasting a wide variety of programs.

Ratings: Surveys to find out the size and type of television audiences watching particular shows during specific times. Information gathered from ratings is used to determine the cost of advertising on each TV show.

Sitcom: A situation comedy, or half-hour comedy show, on TV. A sitcom usually centres on a small group of characters in a specific situation, such as a home or workplace.

Slogan: A snappy, memorable line that helps you remember a product's name. TV viewers see and hear slogans during commercials.

Station: The place that houses the equipment used for transmitting and receiving TV signals.

Stereotype: Standard character type. Stereotypes include the goofy best friend who causes problems, the ugly bad guy, and the dumb blonde.

Storyboard: A kind of detailed comic strip of an entire TV show or commercial that is created before anything is shot. The storyboard sets out what kinds of pictures, sounds, etc., are required, shot by shot.

Stunt: A difficult or dangerous act performed by specially trained actors. TV stunts include car crashes, falls from buildings, and fights.

Sweeps: Ratings sweepstakes. Sweeps take place several times a year – in March, July and November in Canada, and in February, May, July, and November in the U.S. – and are the times when the networks go all-out to attract viewers and receive the highest ratings for their shows.

Syndicate: To sell the rights to show a TV program a limited number of times.

Taped: Recorded on videotape. When a TV program is taped, it can be edited and shown again later. Live TV, on the other hand, is shown to viewers at the same time as it is shot.

V Chip: Viewer control chip. The V Chip is a device that can be programmed to block out certain violent shows or certain levels of TV violence.

Back of the Book

What is "public TV"?

Unlike network television, public television doesn't exist to make money. Commercial networks rely on advertisers' money to pay for their programs and so they tend to produce the kind of programs that have the largest audiences and attract the highest advertising rates. Both the Canadian and American governments established public TV networks that are owned or paid for by the public through taxes and supported by donations from businesses and people who watch public TV. Without the need to make a profit, public TV is able to provide a greater variety of programs, including programs that might never be shown on the networks. Instead of the ads you see on the commercial networks, the American public television network, PBS (Public Broadcasting System), for example, simply announces the corporate sponsors: "Funding for this program was provided by…" and shows the company's logo or name.

(At the time this book was written, the U.S. government was considering disbanding PBS in an attempt to save money. Taxpayers pay less than a dollar a year per person for the privilege of receiving PBS. Many people feel that this is a small price to pay for maintaining such a wide choice of programs. If you are concerned about the future of PBS, write to your government representatives. See page 95.)

Public television in Canada is somewhat different. Canada's public television network, the CBC (Canadian Broadcasting Corporation), was established in the 1930s, first as a radio network, by the Canadian government to protect Canada's unique culture. The CBC ensures that television programs reach all Canadians, no matter how isolated they are. CBC-TV broadcasts programs in both official languages, English and French, as well as in native languages to people in the Canadian North. The CBC does show some American programs because they earn the highest advertising rates and allow the CBC to produce its own shows. The CBC is financed both by taxes and the sale of airtime to advertisers.

Like public television in the U.S., educational TV in Canada has no commercials. Financed by the taxes paid to the provincial governments, Radio Quebec, TVOntario, the Saskatchewan Communications Network, ACCESS Alberta, and the Knowledge Network of the West (KNOW) in British Columbia operate like PBS in the States.

What is a network?

A TV network is a national company that makes and supplies or transmits programs and commercials to a country-wide "network" of local stations linked by satellite. Local stations can't afford to make all their own programs, so they usually show all the network's prime-time shows. In return, the network receives a large audience for their shows and high advertising fees from their advertisers.

The original three networks in the U.S. – NBC (National Broadcasting Company), CBS (Columbia Broadcasting System) and ABC (American Broadcasting Company) – all began as privately owned radio networks in the 1920s. NBC was a creation of RCA (Radio Corporation of America), a company that made lots of money by selling radios. CBS was formed a year later, in 1927, and bought a year after that by William S. Paley, the advertising manager of his family's cigar company, who was greatly impressed by the power of radio ads to double cigar sales in just six months. ABC splintered from NBC and became the third network in 1943. NBC, CBS, and ABC quickly established networks of local stations all across the United States.

In 1986, a brand-new network called Fox was started. Right now, Fox and the other three networks are owned by extremely large companies that also own newspapers, magazines, book publishers, and/or radio stations.

In the States, there are also about 50 cable networks, including MTV, CNN, and Nickelodeon, as well as 10 pay-cable networks. Unlike the four main networks, which pay local stations to show their programs, local cable companies buy programs from the cable network.

In Canada, there are two major English-language networks, CTV (Canadian Television Network) and the CBC (Canadian Broadcasting Corporation). CTV is Canada's only commercial, or privately owned, network, while the CBC is partly owned by Canadian taxpayers. Canada also has three French-language TV networks.

Some of the Canadian specialty channels, including YTV, and pay-TV channels such as The Movie Network, call themselves networks. However, they are different from the "regular" networks. Specialty channels "feed" all their programs to local cable companies across the country. The stations that are part of a regular network have to show only some of the network's programs.

CANADA

The CRTC (Canadian Radio-Television and Telecommunications Commission) is the equivalent of the FCC in the U.S.; it governs radio and television. (It also oversees the telephone companies.) Advertising to children is watched over by the Children's Clearance Committee (CCC), which is part of the Advertising Standards Council (ASC), an organization funded by advertising agencies and the companies that have ads on television and radio and in newspapers and magazines.

The Broadcast Code for Advertising to Children (under 12)
The Advertising Standards Council makes sure that ads to kids follow a special set of rules called the "Broadcast Code for Advertising to Children." The CCC staff must see and approve the final filmed version. If a TV network or station shows an ad that hasn't been cleared by the ASC, and breaks a rule in the Code, the CRTC can take away the broadcaster's licence.

The following are excerpts from the Broadcast Code.
Advertisers must:
1. Make it clear how large a product is by showing it in relation to a person or recognizable other thing
2. Give the product the same amount of time as premiums they're sold with
3. Give clear, thorough information about prices
4. Explain clearly when assembly is required
5. Make it clear when toys are sold separately

Advertisers are not allowed to:
1. Exaggerate
2. Use words like "new" for more than a year
3. Advertise vitamins or drugs
4. Directly recommend that kids buy their product, or ask their parents to
5. Have more than one commercial for the same product during each half-hour period
6. Use well-known characters or famous people to endorse products
7. Suggest that owning this particular product will make you better than other kids
8. Show kids or adults doing risky things with the product

Highlights from The CAB Voluntary Code Regarding Violence in Television Programming, November 1993 (Private Broadcasters)

The Canadian broadcasting authority, the CRTC, decided after much debate to limit the rights of adults to see anything they want in order to protect Canadian kids under 12. The Canadian government encouraged private broadcasters to adopt a voluntary self-regulatory code. The CBSC (Canadian Broadcast Standards Council) of the CAB (Canadian Association of Broadcasters) first developed a voluntary code regarding violence in TV programming in 1987 and updated it in 1993. Broadcasters must follow the code or their licence to broadcast may not be renewed.

"Canadian private broadcasters are publicly endorsing the following principles:
1. that programming containing gratuitous* violence not be telecast,
2. that young children not be exposed to programming which is unsuitable for them,
3. that viewers be informed about the content of programming they choose to watch.

"The depiction of violence within children's programming shall not be so realistic as to threaten young children, to invite imitation, or to trivialize the effects of violent acts.

"Canadian broadcasters shall not air programming which contains gratuitous violence in any form or sanctions, promotes or glamorizes violence."

The Code with Regard to Children's Programming (children being under 12 years old):
"1. …very little violence, either physical, verbal or emotional, shall be portrayed in children's programming.
2. In children's programming portrayed by real-life characters, violence shall only be portrayed when it is essential to the development of character and plot.
3. Animated programming for children, while accepted as a stylized form of story-telling which can contain non-realistic violence, shall not have violence as its central theme, and shall not invite dangerous imitation.
4. Programming for children shall deal carefully with themes which could threaten their sense of security, when portraying, for example: domestic conflict, the death of parents or close relatives, or the death or injury of their pets, street crime or the use of drugs.
5. Programming for children shall deal carefully with themes which could invite children to imitate acts which they see on screen, such as the use of plastic bags as toys, use of matches, the use of dangerous household products as playthings, or dangerous physical acts as climbing apartment balconies or rooftops.
6. Programming for children shall not contain realistic scenes of violence which create the impression that violence is the preferred way,

(*Gratuitous means material which does not play an integral role in developing the plot, character or theme of the material as a whole.)

or the only method to resolve conflict between individuals.

7. Programming for children shall not contain realistic scenes of violence which minimize or gloss over the effects of violent acts. Any realistic depictions shall portray, in human terms, the consequences of that violence to its victims and its perpetrators.

8. Programming for children shall not contain frightening or otherwise excessive special effects not required by the storyline."

With regard to scheduling:
"1. Programming which contains scenes of violence intended for adult audiences shall not be telecast before the late evening viewing period, defined as 9 p.m. to 6 a.m.

5. Broadcasters shall take special precautions to advise viewers of the content of programming intended for adult audiences which is telecast before 9 p.m.

– Promotional material which contains scenes of violence intended for adult audiences shall not be telecast before 9 p.m.

– Advertisements which contain scenes of violence intended for adult audiences, such as those for theatrically presented feature films, shall not be telecast before 9 p.m."

UNITED STATES

Highlights of CARU's Guidelines for Advertising to Children (under 12)

The Children's Advertising Review Unit (CARU) was set up by advertisers to make sure that no ads directed to kids under 12 were misleading or inaccurate. Of the approximately 2000 TV commercials the staff review each month, a handful of advertisements require further examination by a panel of experts – including people from the advertising business and some child psychologists –

who decide whether the ads are honest and fair. If the experts decide that an ad breaks one of their guidelines, the advertiser is asked to change the commercial.

Advertisers don't have to make the change, but CARU does publish a written report of the case, so the advertisers usually do make the changes CARU requests.

Advertisers must:
1. Make sure animation doesn't make something look better or work better than it really does
2. Show the product used in safe ways
3. Be very clear as to what is included and what is not
4. Show snack foods as snacks and not a substitute for a healthy meal
5. Avoid excessively violent or frightening presentations
6. Tell if the product needs to be assembled or needs batteries, or whether batteries must be purchased separately
7. Use celebrities only when they really believe in and use the product
8. Only allow celebrities to endorse a product if they are not usually identified with the product through a related profession

Advertisers are not allowed to:
1. Mislead kids about the size, colour, sound, nutritiousness, or speed of the product
2. Suggest that a product will make them stronger, more popular or smarter
3. Urge kids to ask their parents to buy the product
4. Use words like "now" and "only" to suggest that it's necessary to buy quickly
5. Use animated or human TV characters to promote a product during a kids' program in which that character appears
6. Present premiums (prizes) as more important than the product itself
7. Advertise drugs or vitamins directly to kids

Standards for the Depiction of Violence in Prime-Time Television Programs as issued by ABC, CBS, and NBC in December 1992

In the United States, Congress hasn't ruled against TV violence, although the members have hinted that they will pass a law if the TV makers don't reduce the violence. In response, the three major U.S. networks – ABC, CBS, and NBC – issued a statement in late 1992, promising to limit violence that was excessive and not to show realistic violence in kids' programs:

"1. Conflict and strife are the essence of drama and conflict often results in physical or psychological violence. However, all depictions of violence should be relevant and necessary to the development of character, or to the advancement of theme or plot.

2. Gratuitous or excessive depictions of violence (or redundant violence shown solely for its own sake) are not acceptable.

3. Programs should not depict violence as glamorous, nor as an acceptable solution to human conflict.

4. Depictions of violence may not be used to shock or stimulate the audience.

5. Scenes showing excessive gore, pain or physical suffering are not acceptable.

6. The intensity and frequency of the use of force, and other factors relating to the manner of its portrayal, should be measured under a standard of reasonableness so that the program, on the whole, is appropriate for a home viewing medium.

7. Scenes which may be instructive in nature, e.g., which depict in an imitable manner, the use of harmful devices or weapons, describe readily usable techniques for the commission of crimes, or show replicable methods for the evasion of detection or apprehension, should be avoided. Similarly, ingenious, unique or otherwise unfamiliar methods of inflicting pain or injury are unacceptable if easily capable of imitation.

8. Realistic depictions of violence should also portray, in human terms, the consequences of that violence to its victims and its perpetrators. Callousness or indifference to suffering experienced by victims of violence should be avoided.

9. Exceptional care must be taken in stories or scenes where children are victims of, or are threatened by acts of violence (physical, psychological, or verbal).

10. The portrayal of dangerous behaviour which would invite imitation by children, including portrayals of the use of weapons or implements readily accessible to this impressionable group, should be avoided.

11. Realistic portrayals of violence as well as scenes, images or events which are unduly frightening or distressing to children should not be included in any program specifically designed for that audience.

12. The use of real animals shall conform to accepted standards of humane treatment. Fictionalized portrayals of abusive treatment should be strictly limited to the legitimate requirements of plot development.

13. Extreme caution must be exercised in any themes, plots or scenes which mix sex and violence. Rape and other sexual assaults are violent, not erotic, behaviour.

14. The scheduling of any program, commercial or promotional material, including those containing violent depictions, should take into consideration the nature of the program, its content and the likely composition of the intended audience.

15. Certain exceptions to the foregoing may be acceptable, as in the presentation of material whose overall theme is clearly and unambiguously anti-violent."

YOU CAN MAKE A DIFFERENCE!

Here are the names and addresses of organizations you can write to for more information or to let them know what you think about television violence, advertising, and shows you like and don't like!

If you wish to write a letter to a particular show, or a particular person, please address your letter to that show or person. There is often a different address for each show (depending on the production company). You can also find the show's address on the network Website, or send an e-mail message from the Website.

IN CANADA

Canadian TV Networks

Note: If you're writing about an American TV show that you've seen on a Canadian network or station, write directly to the U.S. network that it came from.

Baton/CTV
9 Channel Nine Court
Toronto, ON M1S 4B5
Website: www.baton.com

CBC (Canadian Broadcasting Corporation)
Audience Relations
P.O. Box 500, Station A
Toronto, ON M5W 1E6
Website: www.cbc.ca   www.cbc4kids.ca

Global Television Network
(CanWest Global System)
Media Relations
81 Barber Greene Road
Don Mills, ON M3C 2A2

YTV Canada
Viewer Relations
64 Jefferson Avenue, Unit 9
Toronto, ON M6K 3H3
Website: www.ytv.com

If you're not happy with your local station's response to your complaint about a violent program, write:

Canadian Broadcast Standards Council (CBSC)
P.O. Box 3265, Station D
Ottawa, ON K1P 6H8
Website: www.cbsc.ca

The CBSC administers four codes: violence, sex-role stereotyping, ethics, and journalistic ethics, and forwards any citizen's complaints to the broadcasters in question, who usually settle directly with whoever has complained.

To complain about a misleading children's advertisement, write to:

Advertising Standards Canada
Children's Advertising Section
Standards Council
350 Bloor Street East, Suite 402
Toronto, ON M4W 1H5
Website: www.canad.com

To complain about inappropriate programming (too much or not enough of one type of program) or anything else, write to:

Secretary-General
CRTC (Canadian Radio-Television and Telecommunications Commission)
Ottawa, ON K1A 0N2
Website: www.crtc.gc.ca

To tell your government representatives what you think about various TV issues such as violence and advertising and to find out what their stand on these issues is, write to:

[Your Member of Parliament]
The House of Commons
Parliament Buildings
Ottawa, ON K1A 0A6
Website: www.parl.gc.ca

For more information about issues regarding television for kids, you can write to:

The Alliance for Children and Television
60 St. Clair Avenue East, Suite 1002
Toronto, ON M4T 1N5
Website: www.act-canada.com

ACT (formerly the Children's Broadcast Institute) is a national, non-profit organization which promotes the interests of children with respect to television. You and your parents may be interested in their parents' guide, Minding the Set! Making Television Work for You and Your Family, *and their multimedia media-literacy guide for parents of young children called* Prime Time Parent.

Coalition for Responsible Television
9405 Sherbrooke East
Montréal, PQ H1L 6P3
Website: www.screen.com/mnet/
eng/med/home/diff/voice.htm

The Coalition has set up a 900 number for Canadians to call to comment on, compliment, or complain about any aspect of Canadian TV. A phone call costs $3; be ready to give your name and address, and the station, date, and time the TV program aired. The Coalition will pass your comment on to the CBSC and the CRTC, if the complaint is within their mandate. If you're under 18, you'll need your parents' permission to call.

Media Awareness Network
Website: www.schoolnet.ca/medianet

Visit this Website to read about how TV and other media are produced and marketed. Find out what kids your age are saying and doing about TV.

IN THE UNITED STATES

American TV Networks

ABC (American Broadcasting Company)
Audience Information
77 West 66th Street
New York, NY 10023
Website: www.abc.com

CBS (Columbia Broadcasting System)
Audience Services
524 West 52nd Street
New York, NY 10019
Website: www.cbs.com

FBC (Fox Broadcasting Company)
Fox Viewer Services
P.O. Box 900
Beverly Hills, CA 90213
Website: www.foxworld.com

NBC (National Broadcasting Company)
Viewer Services
30 Rockefeller Plaza
New York, NY 10112
Website: www.nbc.com

PBS (Public Broadcasting System)
PBS Viewer Mail
1320 Braddock Place
Alexandria, VA 22314-1698
Website: www.pbs.org

Nickelodeon
Viewer Services
1515 Broadway
New York, NY 10036
Website: www.nick.com

To complain about violent TV programs, write to:

Complaints and Investigations Branch
FCC (Federal Communication Commission)
Mass Media Bureau
2025 M St. NW, Room 8210
Washington, DC 20554
Website: www.fcc.gov

To complain about false or misleading TV commercials, write to:

FTC (Federal Trade Commission)
Bureau of Consumer Protection
Washington, DC 20580
Website: www.ftc.gov

CARU (Children's Advertising Review Unit)
Council of Better Business Bureaus, Inc.
845 Third Avenue
New York, NY 10022
Website:
www.bbb.org.advertising/childrensMonitor.html

To tell your government representatives what you think about various TV issues such as violence, advertising, and the proposed cutbacks to PBS, and to find out what their stand is on these issues, write to:

[Your congressperson]
United States House of Representatives
Washington, DC 20515
Website: www.house.gov/writerep

[Your senator]
United States Senate
Washington, DC 20510
Website: www.senate.gov/senator/membmail.html

For more information about issues to do with television for kids, you can write to:

Center for Media Education & Campaign for Kids' TV
1511 K St., NW, Suite 518
Washington, DC 20005
Website: www.cme.org/cme

The Campaign for Kids' TV is committed to improving the quality of children's television, educating the public about the effects of TV, and empowering parents and educators to deal more effectively with the media.

National Foundation to Improve Television
50 Congress Street, Suite 925
Boston, MA 02109

It's not always easy to figure out which company owns the product that's being advertised, and that's where an organization like the National Foundation to Improve Television (FIT) comes in very handy. Kids and their parents can contact FIT to find out what company to write to, as well as its address and a contact name. FIT pushes the FCC, advertisers, and networks to crack down on TV violence.

Zillions Subscription Department
P.O. Box 51777
Boulder, CO 80323-1777

Zillions is a kids' magazine published by Consumers Union, a nonprofit organization established to give consumers the information they need to use their money wisely.

TIPS FOR WRITING EFFECTIVE LETTERS

1. Write as soon as possible after you see the show or ad.
2. Be specific. Tell the person you're writing to exactly what you want them to do.
3. Be personal. Use sentences beginning with the words "I feel…"
4. Ask for an answer.
5. Be brief.
6. Be sure to keep copies of your letters and the answers in case you need them again.

ANSWERS

TV talk, page 11
1. d, 2. a. 3. c. 4. b

How sound effects help you "see," page 40
1. f, 2. e, 3. a, 4. b, 5. d, 6. c

Take a break!, page 57
1. g, 2. f, 3. b, 4. e, 5. d, 6. c, 7. a

Activities

by Chris M. Worsnop

The activities in this chapter will help you learn more about the topics and issues covered in the rest of the book. Activities 12, 35 and 36 were written for parents or teachers, so that they can adapt them for kids, but most were written for kids to read and work on themselves. You might be using this book in your school, in a home-schooling setting, or on your own, just for fun. The activities encourage you to probe, challenge, and extend the ideas in the book with work that is interesting and fun. How about starting a media notebook to use in these activities? It will become a record of your growing media awareness.

I've written a number of books about media education. Some of them are listed in the bibliography on page 110.

❶ Look at the sidebar on page 5. Ask some people you know what it would take to get them to give up TV altogether. Make a poster to show your results.

❷ Make some charts and/or graphs to show the following information about people you know:

✦How many have a TV at home?

✦How many have more than one TV at home?

✦How many have a VCR at home?

✦How many have a video camera at home?

✦How many have any of the above in their own room?

✦How many watch less than one hour of TV a day?

✦How many watch between one and two hours a day?

✦How many watch between two and three hours a day?

✦How many watch between three and four hours a day?

✦How many watch more than four hours a day?

3 Make a list of activities that kids your age enjoy (sports, reading, hobbies, and so on). Make a graph to compare the length of time that different kids spend on TV-watching compared to activities. What do you find?

Do people who spend a lot of time watching TV also spend a lot of time on other things? Do people who have many hobbies spend less time on TV? How many people find lots of time to spend on both TV and activities?

WELCOME TO TV LAND!

4 TV has some standard ways of telling the audience what to expect, such as laugh tracks in a comedy show. In old western movies, the good characters always wore white hats, and the "baddies" always had dark-coloured hats. These devices are called "conventions." Complete the following chart to try your hand at recognizing some other TV conventions.

CONVENTION	EXAMPLE TV SHOW	WHAT THE AUDIENCE EXPECTS
creepy music	*Buffy the Vampire Slayer* (graveyard scene)	to be scared
romantic music		
close-up of a gun		
man with a hat pulled low over his face		
pretty girl catching the eye of a handsome young man		
camera moving in to focus on something falling from a character's pocket		
rain clouds covering the sun		
a door being accidentally left unlocked		
an oil lamp being put down in a barn filled with straw		

5 Use any legal TV video you have to help explain the expression "conventions." ("Legal" video-tapes are copyright-cleared for use in your area. Check the copyright laws where you live to make sure you are not breaking them. If you need help, ask a resource person. Do a Web search on the topic of "video copyright." If in doubt, ask your teacher about Cable-in-the-Classroom.)

Play the tape and be on the lookout for clues that help you know what to expect. Start a report in your TV notebook, beginning with the sentence "I can tell from the first minute or two of a program whether it will be a comedy, a mystery, a romance, or something else . . ." and go on to explain the clues you found in this program.

6 Make a list of your friends' favourite TV shows. Next, list all the characters in those shows. Classify the list of characters in as many ways as you can (for example by gender, age, "goodness," race, wealth, honesty, employment status.) Think about these classifications. What patterns do you see? Which characters appear in more than one list? Are there any kinds of people who never appear on TV? Are there any kinds of people who appear on TV more often than you see them in real life? How many people do you see on TV who are just like you and your friends?

7 Stereotyped, or "standard," characters are common on TV. Write down the names of a few different ones. Next, under each name, write down as many other TV characters as you can think of that belong to the same "standard" character type. At the bottom of each list, write a short definition on the stereotype. (Using examples from the movies, your list might look like this: Luke Skywalker, Robin Hood, Sir Lancelot – brave, handsome, young, supporter of the underdog – "romantic hero.")

8 Answer the question at the top of page 15. Survey some of your friends to find out how much TV they watch each day, and have them answer the same question. Do a written or oral report to explain what you found out. Ask yourself this question as well: "If it turns out that the people who watch a lot of TV are also the people who believe they are going to be victims of crime, does that mean that watching TV makes them believe this? Could there be another cause for this belief?"

9 What is a TV jolt? Along with some friends, read pages 16 and 17 for ideas on jolts. Then take a short section of a video and count the jolts in it. You will probably have to watch it several times to find them all, and you may not always agree over what is or is not a jolt. Which programs would you expect to have the most jolts? Which would have fewer? Why?

10 A "hot switch" is one way that the broadcasters try to make sure you don't change channels at the end of a program. It means going directly from the end of one show into the start of the next without a break for commercials. Make a short list of other ways that broadcasters try to keep you tuned in.

11 Write your explanations of each of the following terms in your TV notebook. (You'll find the answers in "Welcome to TV Land!")

• convention　　　　• stereotype　　　　• jolt　　　　• hot switch　　　　• teaser

BEHIND THE SCENES WITH LYNNE CARROW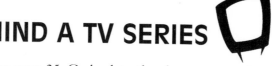

12 Some children have had the experience of auditioning for TV shows or commercials, or have taken courses to prepare them for work as TV actors or models. Try to arrange for one of these students to give a talk to your class about their experiences. Prepare plenty of questions in advance.

13 Have you ever thought that a certain actor would be perfect in a certain role? Talk to some people your own age to gather examples. Do you all agree? Why or why not? Try to answer the following questions:

✦Do some actors specialize in playing stereotyped characters? If so, which actors? Which characters?

✦Are some actors able to play many kinds of characters? Which actors? What were the parts they played? How were they different from each other?

14 On page 21, Lynne Carrow says: "People don't want to watch real life on TV." Hold a debate on this topic.

15 Add your explanations of the expression "typecasting" to your TV notebook.

THE STORY BEHIND A TV SERIES

16 Look at the sidebar on page 25. Go back to the charts you made earlier listing your favourite shows. Check them out to see if the claim in the sidebar is true for you and your friends.

17 When XYZ TV is testing a show, why are they interested in how much money people in the audience make? Make up a list of questions you would like to see included in the testing of new TV shows. Write down why you think each question is important.

18 Use the sidebar at the bottom of page 26 as a guide for writing a group letter to a TV station or network about one of your favourite shows. (Check "Back of the Book" for addresses.) You will find guidelines for letter-writing in some language arts textbooks and in some word-processing software programs.

19 Work with two or three other kids to make up a perfect night of TV, with a schedule that creates no conflicts for anyone in your group. Start with a real evening's TV schedule and rearrange the programs to your liking. Have one member of the group keep track of all the different kinds of difficulties you had in agreeing on the schedule. (See pages 27-28.)

20 Work with a partner to write a newspaper article called "Who Pays for TV?" Explain how TV producers get the money to pay for the programs they make, and how the people who pay for the programs get their money back.

If $4 a minute is the going cost-per-thousand (CPM) rate for advertising, how much would a two-minute commercial cost during the Olympics, which had 60 million viewers? ({60,000,000 /1000} x $4 x 2 = $480,000!) How do advertisers get back the money they spend on advertising?

㉑ Think about what the last two activities have taught you, and discuss the meaning of the saying "TV is free entertainment."

㉒ Add your explanations of these expressions to your TV notebook:
- CPM
- Pilot
- Prime-time
- Ratings
- Sweep
- Sitcom
- Syndicated show

BEHIND THE SCENES WITH GOODY GERNER

㉓ How would you decide whether a TV show for kids was good enough to put on the air, *before* you spent a lot of money on it? Talk to some friends and write down your ideas. Then, if possible, hold a discussion to find the best five ideas from different groups. Then read the interview with Goody Gerner to see if your ideas are the same as the ones used by the professionals.

㉔ What is a "focus group"? How do focus groups work? Make up an idea for a kids' TV show. Write down your ideas and an outline of what would happen in the first episode. Then, form a focus group from other kids and test the idea, the same way Goody Gerner did with real TV shows. Keep notes and a tape recording of your focus-group sessions. Use the suggestions from the group to improve your proposal for the TV show. Use another focus group if you have the time, and do another round of changes to your proposal. You might even consider sending the finished proposal to a TV producer or network.

㉕ Add your explanations of these expressions to your TV notebook:
- focus group
- testing shows

WHAT DO YOU SEE ON TV?

To do your work on this chapter and also some of the later ones, it would be a good idea to collect some magazines, newspapers, and comic strips that you can cut up. If you have access to a video camera or a still camera (Polaroid is best because you get to see the pictures right away), get permission to use it. For some of the exercises, you will need toilet-paper tubes and paper-towel tubes. If you can find tubes longer than paper-towel tubes, so much the better. These can be the lenses of your imaginary camera. The short tube will be the wide-angle lens, the longer tube will give you medium shots, and the longest tube will be a close-up, or telephoto, lens. To make the tubes more like camera lenses, cut out a rectangular cardboard frame and paste it over the end away from your eye, so that what you see through it will have the same shape as a TV picture.

Since the camera has only one lens, whereas you have two eyes, you must always close one eye when looking through your cardboard lenses.

26 Use a video camera, still camera, or cardboard tube to look around you. Move your camera around to compose some "shots" that:

✦ make a little kid look bigger than a big kid. (How did you do it?)

✦ make a small group of kids look like a crowd. (How did you do it?)

✦ make one kid in a crowded room look as if he or she is the only one there. (How did you do it?)

✦ make something that is small look very important. (How did you do it?)

✦ make it clear that a kid is being looked at from the point of view of an adult. (How did you do it?)

✦ make it clear that a kid is anxious about the time showing on the clock. (How did you do it?)

✦ make it clear that something a kid is holding is more important to look at than the kid. (How did you do it?)

27 Tell a story with pictures. Either draw a storyboard, make a comic strip (almost the same thing as a storyboard), shoot a series of photographs using a Polaroid camera, or make a short video. (Be sure to use establishing shots, medium shots and close-ups – see pages 43-44.) Show:

✦ how to get from the classroom door to a desk in the far corner of the room.

✦ a very small, timid student taking her book to the very tall, domineering teacher.

✦ a certain student in the class looking small and nervous to the teacher who sits a long way off, but big and confident to another student who sits at the next desk.

✦ a student in a group of ten students, but make her look either like part of a larger crowd or as though she were alone.

✦ a big kid looking smaller than a little kid, even though the big kid is closer to the camera.

28 Use camera tricks to make up a short scene of your own, in which the camera makes the viewer see something differently from how it actually happened.

29 Tell a story with sound and music only. Take a tape recorder and make a story, using only sounds, but without words or dialogue. Play your tape for some friends and see if they can recognize your story. Use them as a focus group to help you make improvements to your sound-effects story.

30 Become a foley artist. Take some common objects and create sound effects like the ones on TV (a door banging, leaves rustling, a log fire crackling). Tape-record your results. Play your tape for other people and challenge them to tell how you made the sound effects.

31 Make up some visual stories of your own by cutting up newspaper cartoons and pasting the pictures together in a new order to tell a new story. Ask your friends to tell a different story using the same pictures. (The National Film Board of Canada short video *Sequence and Story* would be a good resource to use along with this activity.)

32 When TV makes something look or sound different from what it really is, we call it "a construction." It is a construction because TV has put it together, or "constructed" it, in a special way that never existed in real life. Read this chapter again and count all the examples of TV constructions. Check your own list against someone else's to make sure you caught all the examples. (A good resource for this activity is the chapter "The Camera Always Lies" in my book *Screening Images: Ideas for Media Education*.)

33 Write a journal entry on the topic of TV constructions, answering the questions below:

✦How surprised were you to find out about TV constructions?

✦How much of it did you already know? How did you come to know it?

✦Is all of TV a construction? Is there ever anything on TV that is not constructed?

✦Will your understanding of construction on TV change the way you watch TV?

✦Will it spoil your enjoyment of TV?

34 This chapter contains many new terms for you to explain in your TV notebook. You can do these alone or share the work with someone else. Use examples from newspapers, magazines, or comic strips to paste in your notes as illustrations of some of these terms:

• point of view	• frame	• shot	• angle
• camera distance	• sound effects	• foley artist	• storyboard
• high-angle	• low-angle	• eye-level	• long-shot
• establishing shot	• medium shot	• close-up	• extreme close-up
• laugh track	• sweetening	• quick cuts	• editing
• flashback	• hand-held camera	• you-are-there	• construction

BEHIND THE SCENES WITH JOHN NELLES

John Nelles' first speech in this interview tells us how important it is to understand camera placement and how the camera "sees." The next activities provide some practical experiences to illustrate Nelles' points.

35 Pick any section of dramatic (that is, fictional) TV or film, and play "where's the camera?" For every scene in the section, draw a diagram to show where the actors and the camera are located. You might have to draw both a floor plan and a side view to explain everything about the camera placement. Which scenes were the hardest to figure out? Why? For an even bigger challenge, try playing "where's the camera?" with TV commercials or music videos.

36 In some programs, children are never seen except from an adult eye-level. In other shows, because the camera is placed at the kids' own eye level, the world and the kids themselves look more natural to other kids. Show some TV programs that feature kids. Have the kids draw diagrams to show how the eye level of the camera in these programs can make them look natural or "inferior."

37 Go out-of-doors to a playground or sports field, or work inside a large room like a gym, for this activity. Have the group answer these questions:

How can you make objects look different

✦by placing the camera in various positions?

✦by using the long or short lens tube?

✦by moving the camera as you look through the lens?

38 Look up these expressions in a book or on the Internet:

• parallax   • binocular vision

39 Watch some episodes of TV programs that might be called violent. Study them to see where and how the violent actions have been made safe for the actors. (For instance, when a stunt performer falls from a roof, you either do not see the landing, or sometimes see that the fall ends in a pile of cardboard boxes which collapse on impact. When you do not see the end of the fall, that is because the actor was falling into a special soft mattress or a net. When the fall ends in a pile of empty boxes, the boxes have been specially constructed to break the fall safely.) After giving the shows a close second look, make a display using models and/or diagrams to explain what you see.

40 Sometimes a person being interviewed does not answer the interviewer's questions, but instead "answers" another question that was never asked. Can you find a place where John Nelles does this with his interviewer? (Look on page 51.) Why do you think people do this in interviews? Listen to some other interviews and try to find more examples of the same thing.

41 Make up some interview topics and take turns pretending to be the interviewer or the person being interviewed. When it's your turn, try answering questions different from the ones you've been asked.

42 Add your explanations of these expressions to your TV notebook:

• stunt   • choreographer   • media violence   • safety

• candy glass   • computer-generated special effects   • consequences

"WE'LL BE RIGHT BACK AFTER THESE MESSAGES"

43 What do you do during commercials? Ask several people this question and make up a chart or series of graphs to explain to your friends or classmates what you found out.

44 "Commercials pay for most of the programs you watch." Which TV channels do *not* carry commercials? How do those channels pay for their programs? What differences are there between the programs on these non-commercial channels and the ones on the commercial channels? Make a poster to show the differences you have found.

45 When you're watching a TV show and you see any of the following, you are seeing "product placement."

+ a character drinking a certain brand of cola, with the label held in clear view
+ someone driving a certain kind of car in every episode of a program
+ a character wearing a recognizable brand of clothing or shoes
+ a scene taking place in a real-life fast-food restaurant

The products have been deliberately placed there for you to see and recognize. During one evening of TV viewing, keep a notebook of product-placement messages you have seen in the programs you watched. (Remember that product placement comes in the program, not in the commercials.) Do you think product placement persuades people to buy certain products? If you wanted to avoid it, what could you do?

46 Infomercials are usually aimed at adults. Can you think of any infomercials that are aimed at audiences your age? Maybe the cartoons that feature characters based on toys or other products are really infomercials. Maybe music video shows are infomercials. What do you think?

Look at the section called Some TV Tricks of the Trade on pages 54-55. It explains the advertising techniques of:

• repetition   • SFX   • come-ons   • language-baiting   • celebrity endorsement

47 Watch one episode of a program and analyze two of the commercials you see to find as many examples of these techniques as you can. Did you find any other techniques? Discuss what you found out in either a written or an oral report.

48 Since you started reading this chapter, how many times have you heard someone say advertising does not influence them? Do a survey. Pick a kind of product (for example toys, clothes, shoes, or electronics) and ask around to find out how many people actually own or use things they have seen advertised. For instance, what proportion of the group buys no-name soft drinks as opposed to brand-name soft drinks? How many own nationally advertised toys and sports equipment, and how many own other kinds? How many own all new things, and how many buy second-hand or hand-me-down things? Use the information in the sidebar on page 56 to calculate how much each person spends indirectly supporting advertising. (You can also use the numbers from Calling All Shoppers! on page 61.)

49 Start a collection of "commercials I love and hate." Describe them in your media journal and add a few comments about each one to explain what you particularly like or dislike.

50 Play the role of "watchdog" and look for commercials that you think come close to breaking the rules listed on pages 89-92. Using the advice and information on page 58, write a letter about a commercial that makes you mad. Write another letter about a commercial that you think deserves praise.

51 Hold a debate about whether TV commercials should be allowed a regular place in classrooms. Talk to some older kids in schools where Channel One News is operating and find out how it's working out. (The Canadian Youth News Network is still at the planning stage.)

52 Add your explanations of these expressions to your TV notebook:

- commercial
- infomercial
- CRTC/FCC
- endorsement
- stretching the truth
- watchdog
- disclaimer
- brand loyalty

BEHIND THE SCENES WITH REBECCA GREENSTEIN AND DALIA ROTSTEIN

53 Find some TV commercials that base their claims on experiments. Get the addresses for the makers of the products advertised in the commercials, and do what Rebecca and Dalia did:

✦Write to the manufacturers for information.

✦See if you can duplicate the experiments.

✦Write again to the manufacturers to tell them your results.

✦Write a report on your project for a science fair and/or local newspaper.

54 Rebecca says: "I think people should look at TV advertising a lot more critically and question everything they see and are told. You really have to go and find out yourself." Make a list of ways you could be more critical of TV ads.

55 Make up a skit in which someone plays the part of a commercial, and others ask it "critical questions."

56 Write a story or play to describe what might happen to TV if there were no ads.

57 Add your explanations of these expressions to your TV notebook:

- face value
- question everything
- critical

FIST FIGHTS, SHOOTOUTS, BLOOD AND GORE

58 Before you can discuss violence on TV, you need to define what violence is. Some people think that any form of disrespect is a form of violence. (See "Behind the Scenes with Virginie Larivière," page 80.) Other people would count only physically harmful actions as violence. Others again would say that it all depends on how it is shown. What do you think?

✦Is a "play punch" in the schoolyard violent?

✦Is calling names violent?

✦Is making fun of someone violent?

✦Is violence only physical?

59 Write a personal note in your TV journal listing some violent actions, scenes or programs you have seen on TV. Next, explain why you think these are examples of violence. Then compare your entry with someone else's to see where you agree and disagree about the definition of violence.

60 Think of a TV show you have seen that ended in violence. Could the story have ended without violence? How? Think about negotiation, compromise, mediation, and the use of the law and the courts as alternatives to fighting and killing. Make up two new endings for the TV show you watched.

61 Think of all the TV shows you have seen where the endings have *not* been violent. How did those shows end? Which shows always try to be non-violent? Which ones always seem to be violent? Which ones do you like the most? Why? Write your answer in your journal. (In answering this last question, you must give real reasons, not just reasons like "Because I like it," or "Because it's good.")

62 Conduct a survey to find out such things as:

✦how many killings you see in an evening's TV-watching

✦how many killings are reported on average in your daily newspaper

✦who the people are who get killed in TV shows (note their age, gender, race, and social status)

✦who the people are who never or rarely get killed on TV

What do your survey results teach you about the way TV shows are written?

63 Reread the section on page 16 about "jolts" and prepare a short talk about how violence on TV is connected to the idea of jolts.

64 Use a cassette recorder to interview as many kids as you can about how they think they've been affected by violence on TV. A few sample questions:

✦How many of them believe they've been made more violent by watching violent TV?

✦How many of them think they've been made more aggressive?

✦How many believe they've been made more afraid of violence?

✦How many believe they're more likely to see violence as a way of solving problems?

✦How many believe they haven't been changed by it at all?

Ask every kid you talk to for examples to back up what they tell you. Edit your tape to make a radio documentary on what kids think about TV violence.

65 Do you have a friend who is never violent? Interview this friend to find out if he or she has ever watched violence on TV. Talk together to try to answer the question of why some people can watch violence on TV and not be affected by it.

66 Get permission to work with a class in school, and show the beginning of a fictional film or TV show on videotape. Pick a story with a good conflict in it that could be resolved either by violence or in some other way. Stop the tape before the ending and ask the students to predict how the show will end. Classify their answers as violent or non-violent. What conclusions can you draw from your results? (Choose or create a play or skit to substitute for the videotape. Repeat the experiment with a different class, performing or reading out the piece you have chosen or created. Compare the results from the two experiments. How do you explain the similarities or differences?)

67 Hold a debate on the topic "People who are violent in real life would be violent even if there were no TV."

68 Write an explanation of the word "gratuitous." Then write about some TV shows you have seen where there was violence that was gratuitous, and about some others, where you thought the violence was not gratuitous. Compare your work with someone else's. Do the two of you agree? Why or why not?

69 What might make people violent besides TV? Talk and think about these questions and then write a story about why a kid your age was or was not influenced by violence on TV.

70 Write letters to local TV stations or cable channels to tell them about the programs you like and dislike, depending on how the shows approach violence. Send copies of your letters to your local newspaper for the readers' letters column. Use the advice on page 71 for contacting your national broadcasting-standards agency if you are not satisfied with the replies to your first letter.

71 Nowadays we use TV as our main entertainment. What did people in the past do for entertainment? (Research colonial North America, ancient Rome, revolutionary France, Victorian England, medieval Europe, and the Incan and Mayan civilizations.) Write a short report or prepare a talk on the level of violence in popular entertainment at different times in history.

72 "If it bleeds, it leads." This has been the policy that many broadcasters used in the past to select items for the news. Check out your local broadcasts to see which ones are still beginning their news programs with stories about violence. Which ones have changed to a different, "family sensitive" approach? (See pages 75-76.) Send letters to your local TV stations to let them know what you think of their news policies. Always give examples of actual stories to back up your opinions.

73 Write an "editorial" on one of the following topics:

✦The V Chip is the answer to the problem of TV violence.

✦The V Chip will limit children's freedom of speech.

✦The V Chip will help parents to protect children.

✦Parents will need their children's help to program the V Chip.

✦The V Chip may help us avoid watching violence, but it may not change the violence in society.

74 Add your explanations of these expressions to your TV notebook:

- channel surfing
- aggressive
- consequences
- gratuitous
- CRTC/FCC
- family-sensitive
- V Chip

BEHIND THE SCENES WITH VIRGINIE LARIVIÈRE

75 Search the files in a library or on the Internet for newspaper and magazine coverage of Virginie Larivière's petition. (Look at material dating from November–December, 1992.) Write and/or videotape a short TV news report about Virginie, using the information and pictures you find.

76 Write the outline of a story for a movie-of-the-week about Virginie Larivière and her petition.

77 Act out a debate between Virginie Larivière and John Nelles on the subject of TV violence.

78 Think of a subject you feel strongly enough about to create a petition. Make a written plan for doing this, listing all the work you would have to do, and all the details you would have to look after.

79 Add your explanations of these expressions to your TV notebook:

• petition   • humiliate   • influence

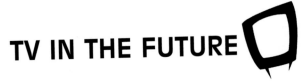

TV IN THE FUTURE

80 Write a story about all the things you would like to see in the future of TV. Go overboard! Use your imagination!

81 If you had to pay each time you watched a show, what difference would that make to the way you watch TV? Write a skit about a family trying to decide what to watch on TV when everything has a cost.

82 Based on the idea "You might see your own veterinarian advertising on the Chihuahua Channel!", make up a list of ads you might see in the future. (For example, you could write about your older brother advertising as a caddy on the local golf channel.)

83 Add your explanations of these expressions to your TV notebook:

• 500-channel universe   • digital   • compressed   • interactive

Resources

The Media Awareness Network at:
http://www.screen.com/mnet/eng
This outstanding Canadian site has regularly updated pages for teachers, parents and children, together with links to numerous other sites.

The Media Literacy Online Project of the University of Oregon at:
http://interact.uoregon.edu/MediaLit/HomePage
This American site is very comprehensive and informative. It is linked to many other major media education sites.

Adbusters Culture Jammers Headquarters at:
http://www.adbusters.org/adbusters/main.html
This site gives anti-consumerist examples of the advertising counter-culture.

KIDS FIRST at:
http://www.cqcm.org/kidsfirst/html/res.htm
This is a page listing a wealth of other resources: magazines, books, pamphlets and newsletters about kids and media.

Theatre Books at:
http://www.theatrebooks.com
This is the best site in Canada for ordering media education materials.

The Center for Media Literacy at:
http://www.medialit.org
This site is good for general information about media education, and for ordering media education materials in the US.

The Center for Children and Technology at:
http://www.edc.org/CCT/ccthome/outpost/index.html
This is the media education page in the CCT website.

The Community Learning Network, Open School Open Learning Agency at:
http://www.etc.bc.ca/tdebhome/themes/media_violence.html
This page contains multiple links to other sites all related to media and violence.

The National Telemedia Council at:
www.ntelemedia@aol.com
The National Telemedia Council is one of the best American sites for media literacy teachers.

Anderson, Neil; Carreiro, Paul; Dede Sinclair et al. *Responding to Media Violence: Starting Points for Classroom Practice*. North York, ON: The Metropolitan Toronto School Board, 1996.

Axelrod, Lauryn. *TV-Proof Your Kids: A Parent's Guide to Safe and Healthy Viewing*. Secaucus NJ: Citadel Press, 1997.

Bianculli, David. *Teleliteracy: Taking Television Seriously*. New York: Continuum, 1994.

Buckingham, David. *Children Talking Television: The Making of Television Literacy*. London: The Falmer Press, 1993.

Buckingham, David. *Watching Media Learning: Making Sense of Media Education*. London: The Falmer Press, 1990.

Chen, Milton. *The Smart Parent's Guide to Kids' TV*. San Francisco: KQED, 1994

De Gaetano, Gloria, and Bander, Kathleen. *Screen Smarts: A Family Guide to Media Literacy*. New York: Houghton Mifflin, 1996.

Worsnop, Chris M. *Assessing Media Work*. Mississauga: Wright Communications, 1996.

Worsnop, Chris M. *Popular Culture (ISSUES Series)*. Toronto: McGraw Hill Ryerson, 1994.

Worsnop, Chris M. *Screening Images: Ideas for Media Education*. Mississauga: Wright Communications, 1994.

INDEX

Acknowledgements

Special thanks are due to the following people, all of whom were exceedingly generous with their time and expertise:

Julie T. Hoover, ABC; Jeffrey Kofman, CBC; Nancy Carr, CBS; Reg McGuire, CHCH-TV; Jane Welowszki, CTV; Sandra Puglielli, Global; Ronit Greenstein, PBS; David Way and Mike Jackson, TVO; Tracy Flett, WTN; Michelle Gare, YTV.

For specific assistance with the sections on TV programming: Norene Lowe, Nielsen Marketing Research, Canada; the staff of Nielsen Media Research U.S.; Gail Morrell, CTV; Steve Barone, FCC; Lise Plouffe, CRTC.

For specific assistance with the chapter on TV advertising: Susan Burke, Canadian Advertising Foundation; Pat Beatty, Telecaster; Elizabeth Lascoutx, CARU; Toby Levin, FTC; Michael F. Jacobson, Ph.D., The Center for Science in the Public Interest; Brenda Gaze, Canadian Recording Industry Association.

For specific assistance with the chapter on TV violence: Joanna Santa Barbara, MD; Carole Lieberman, MD, Media Psychiatrist, UCLA Neuro-Psychiatric Institute; Tara Rogan, CBSC; William Abbott, National Foundation to Improve Television; George Gerbner, Dean Emeritus, Annenberg School for Communication; Tim Collings, Simon Fraser University.

For specific assistance with the chapter on TV in the future: Ruth DeSouza, Director of New Product Development, Rogers Cablesystems.

For assistance with the revisions to the second edition: Arlene Moscovitch; Professor Clive Vanderburgh, School of Radio and Television Arts, Ryerson Polytechnic University; Kelly Sercombe and Trina McQueen, Discovery Channel; Susannah Stern, Park Doctoral Fellow, University of North Carolina, Chapel Hill; John Earnhardt, The National Association of Broadcasters; George Gerbner, Dean Emeritus, Annenberg School for Communication, University of Pennsylvania.

And special thanks to Rick Wilks for believing in this book, Debora Pearson for creating order, Brian Bean and Lorraine Tuson for their inspired design and illustrations, Karen Millyard for her patience, perseverance and good humour, Lorraine Greey for teaching me everything I know about making books, Tom Best for his generous and invaluable advice, and Marilyn Ortwein and her grade five class at Rolling Meadows Public School.